THE BEST

ABOUT NUTRITION AND HEALTH

*Simple ways to nurture your health and
avoid the habits that keep you
from living a long and happy life.*

DOROTHY ZIEGLER, R.D.

Printed in Victoria, Canada

National Library of Canada Cataloguing in Publication Data

Ziegler, Dorothy, 1975-
      The best darn book about nutrition and health /
Dorothy Ziegler.
Includes bibliographical references.
ISBN 1-55395-560-9
      I. Title.
RA776.Z53 2003   613   C2003-900135-0

TRAFFORD

This book was published *on-demand* in cooperation with Trafford Publishing.
On-demand publishing is a unique process and service of making a book available for retail sale to the public taking advantage of on-demand manufacturing and Internet marketing. **On-demand publishing** includes promotions, retail sales, manufacturing, order fulfilment, accounting and collecting royalties on behalf of the author.

Suite 6E, 2333 Government St., Victoria, B.C. V8T 4P4, CANADA

Phone	250-383-6864	Toll-free	1-888-232-4444 (Canada & US)
Fax	250-383-6804	E-mail	sales@trafford.com
Web site	www.trafford.com	TRAFFORD PUBLISHING IS A DIVISION OF TRAFFORD

HOLDINGS LTD.

Trafford Catalogue #02-1276   www.trafford.com/robots/03-1276.html

10   9   8   7   6   5   4   3   2   1

This book is dedicated to the loving memory
of my Aunt Norma.

She was a person who made everyone feel special.

The author thanks and recommends these services:

Bleu Cotton Photography
www.bleucotton.com
949-574-1900

Summer Allen at International Hair Systems
www.internationalhairsystems.com
Tustin, CA
714-505-3667

Jenny Warner at Desa European Salon
Costa Mesa, CA
949-645-0311

Nancy Clark, M.S., R.D.
Brookline, MA
www.nancyclarkrd.com

Merrin Folender, R.D.
Los Angeles, CA
merrin@earthlink.net

Johanna Donnenfield, M.S., R.D.
Scottsdale, AZ
auntieyod@msn.com

Don Mankie, R.D.
Salem, VA

Dmankie@lewisgaleclinic.com

Theresa DeLorenzo, R.D.
Tdel8952@postoffice.uri.edu

Dr. Susan Shapiro, R.D.
DrSuShap@pacbell.net

Amber Pawlowski, R.D.
La Jolla, CA
ampawlowski@yahoo.com

Barbara Beznos, R.D., L.D.
Integrated Nutrition, LLC.
Farmington Hills, MI
rds@integratednutrition.com

ACKNOWLEDGEMENTS

I send a loving thank you to my wonderful husband, Brian Ziegler, for encouraging me to pursue my aspirations. I feel honored to have a man like you in my life. Thank you for your care, intense work, and making me a very happy wife!

Thank you to my parents for helping me through my education. You have been extremely supportive in my career as a dietitian. I cherish all of our memories we hold as a family.

I would also like to thank my four editors, Kimberly Tessmer, R.D., L.D., Heather Kangas, Dyann Warrington, and Kimberly Wolfe. Thank you to my professors at Eastern Michigan University who taught me the facts about nutrition, Alice Jo Rainville, Ph. D., R.D., Debbie Silverman, M.S., R.D., FADA, and Polly Buchanan, Ph. D., R.D.. Thank you to my sisters, Heidi and Lindsay, and my best friends Kathy, Heather and Dyann for listening to my nutrition ideas and cheering for me!

Last but not least, thank you for investing in this book. I look forward to helping you reach your ultimate nutritional health and fitness level.

CONTENTS

THE BEST DARN BOOK

ABOUT NUTRITION AND HEALTH

INTRODUCTION

There is mass misunderstanding of nutrition in the world today – especially in America. Many people listen to nutrition and fitness advice from unreliable sources. These people that listen to bad advice, often become fatter, more obsessive, unhappy and unhealthy. You should realize these people know just as much about nutrition as you do. You will become healthier and fit when you *stop* obsessing about what you eat.

This book will teach how vital fat is in the diet and how it's bad to refrain from it. Instead of learning what expensive supplement will support your body the best, you will learn that no supplement supports your body like food does. You'll realize that a lot of the nutrition "hype" marketed through the media and heard through your friends and family is exactly just that…hype! You'll also see how complex nutrition isn't. It is complex in the chemistry and nutrient metabolic pathways. But it is not complex in terms of *good* and *bad*.

I dropped extra weight, became less obsessed and more muscular from my dietetics education and experience. I feel proud of my health. I want to share this marvelous feeling with you. I am not healthy from a "super pill", a new and improved fitness gadget, or from eating no carbohydrates and sugar. I will provide you with the information and motivation to take you where you have never been before. I have included my best from years of counseling patients with all different types of nutrition, fitness and health issues.

Read this book and incorporate what you learn. You can read one chapter and use what you discover to change your health habit. Focus on that one chapter until you've made it a good habit in your life. Then move on to the next chapter and build on to your new lifestyle. Each chapter takes less than ten minutes to read. Before you know it, you'll feel fabulous. You will want to share these health secrets with your friends and family too.

My goal for you is to reach your optimal health. That doesn't mean that you're going to eat, exercise and think just like me. However, it means that you develop a healthy attitude to help you create a body you are proud to live in. So as we begin our journey together, I want you to set your goals higher than you think you can accomplish. The further your aspirations, the further you will take yourself. I am confident that you will experience self-actualization in health. You will revert back to the healthy instincts you were born with. Go get 'em!

- Dorothy Ziegler, R.D.

1.

BE DISCIPLINED

Losing weight is not easy. Working out most days of the week is not always fun. Ordering the fish tacos as opposed to the beef chimichanga can be challenging. Giving up one hour of television or internet surfing per day can be torture. What makes some people choose the healthy option while others continuously opt for the latter? It's discipline!

One way to combat tempting food or the desire to skip exercise is to remember how it feels to be at an undesirable weight. Remembering feelings of pain, rude comments and bad photos can help make you more disciplined.

You don't always have to use negative thoughts. You can also use positive motivation. Imagine what it will be like when you meet your goal weight. Sounds exciting, doesn't it? Or the thought of fitting into your favorite jeans again, YES! The confidence that you will gain is remarkable. There will be those who doubt you can make a change. Proving them wrong is an astonishing feeling!

Discipline is a large component of being nutritionally and physically fit. In a recent poll done by the Calorie Control Council, men and women were asked what their reason was for not being able to lose weight. Forty-one percent of women and twenty-eight percent of men attributed it to lack of self-discipline.

We know what the right thing to do is. But why don't we do it? The number of people exercising after the New Year is great. But where do they go by the end of January? It never fails. The same people are back in April just in time for bathing suit season! The gym is like a ghost town in December. If you are going to exercise, you need to make it a regular part of your weekly, monthly and yearly schedule. It is even possible and very beneficial to squeeze in a workout during the holiday season.

Think about one area of your life in which you are very proud of how disciplined you are. Is this where you concentrate most of your attention? For example, maybe you are extremely focused on your work. It is important to balance your life. You need to develop the skill to be focused in other areas of your life such as exercise. Channel some of this energy to the other aspects of your life that you lack discipline. You will find a deeper sense of satisfaction.

2.

WORKOUTS... FUN?

How could the two words possibly be in the same sentence? Working out and fun just do not go together. And those people that say, "I love aerobics, it's so fun!" or "My morning jog is my favorite time of the day," they must be lying! Right? Wrong! Workouts can be very fun. The challenging part is finding a workout that suits you. Don't feel guilty because you can't learn to like jogging.

I had a friend once who joined me on various sorts of activities. After an all day hike together, he expressed how much he needed to work out. He couldn't figure out when he was going to fit it in nor did he really want to. I looked at him quixotically and said, "What do you mean get a work out in? What do you think we just did? Hiking *is* a work out!" He thought the only way to work out was being underneath a bar full of iron plates.

Many people view working out as having to be grueling, repetitive and within the confinement of a gym. This is exactly why fun workouts are an oxymoron.

Have you ever performed the same activity day after day without much variation? It may have been fun at first but less appealing soon after. The same goes for working out.

Think back to the days as a kid when playing tag was fun. Maybe little league was your passion! I bet you didn't realize you were working out during those times. They were fun ways of working out. That's why you didn't grasp the fact that you were actually exercising.

So change that thought in your head that a work out has to be grueling to be considered as exercise. Begin brainstorming of various activities that may be fun for you. Try learning a new sport each year. Throughout the year you can perfect your skill. You will be getting your exercise in at the same time. Play tennis with your spouse or companion. You will be spending valuable time together. You can even do a nightly activity, such as swing dancing. Couple's dancing is great bonding! Here are some other great ideas:

Snow Skiing	Ice Skating	Snorkeling
Water Skiing	Basketball	Bowling
Hiking	Tennis	Gardening
Kayaking	Dancing	Frisbee
Water Polo	Golf	Karate
Volleyball	Racquet Ball	Gymnastics
Badminton	Biking	Softball
Surfing	Rollerblading	Hockey

Working out doesn't have to be three miles on the treadmill everyday. There is so much more workout opportunities out there than that! Find fun and forget about working out even though you really are!

3.

ARE YOU REALLY HAPPY?

Happiness is produced by different stimuli for different people. For some, hearing rock music makes them happy while for others it causes a twinge of pain. Becoming engaged for some is happiness while for others it causes fear. Some people have no concern with being overweight but it can make others depressed and worrisome. Are you happy with your physical health? This is what matters most.

While the media bombards us with images of what makes happiness, it is important to not let this control our contentment. Each person's body is healthy at different levels of fitness, thinness, fatness, etc. For example, I have a client we'll call her Thea. Thea has established her own body happiness. At one point she forced herself to be very thin. Her body felt weak and tired. She didn't feel attractive and she hated depriving herself of the food that she loves. She was not eating a balanced diet. Some people can eat a healthy and well balanced diet and still be very thin. Thea's body is different. Her body doesn't function correctly when she goes below 123 pounds. Her body fat percentage is too low. Thea feels the healthiest between 125 – 130 pounds. This is Thea's happy weight range. You have your own range.

Think about the weight where your body feels happiest and healthiest. Consider all factors such as health measures (cholesterol levels, blood pressure), mental happiness, energy level and self-confidence. Remember a time in your life when you felt great! This is most likely your optimal weight range. Now consider how you achieved that weight range. Can you incorporate those habits back into your life? Perhaps this is the key to becoming happy again!

4.

EATING HEALTHY IS LIKE BUDGETING MONEY

I have several clients who proclaim to be aces at budgeting money. On the contrary, they are not so good at eating healthy. Eating healthy is like budgeting money.

Dee is planning for her sister's wedding. The wedding is seven months away. She estimates how much money she will have to save each month to cover the costs. Weddings can be expensive. She calculates that she will need $700. Thus she will need to save $100 a month.

Likewise, one must budget food the same way. It may not be desirable to watch carefully what you eat. If you don't, you'll likely gain pounds. Plan for the week ahead of you. Let's pretend *you* have a wedding to attend on Saturday. At weddings you usually enjoy a glass of champagne, appetizers, a glass of wine and a piece of cake. Think about how many calories are in the meal you plan to consume. Be aware of the hidden calories in great tasting catered food.

You are probably wondering how you could afford to eat all that while trying to lose weight. It's simple! You will budget your week's worth of eating. Allowing yourself to have a piece of cake is definitely a grand idea if you really want it. But make that your sugar-laden dessert of the week. During the week choose low fat desserts such as fresh berries or a banana. As for the dinner, enjoy every bite without feeling guilt by choosing lower fat options earlier in the day. For example replace your bran muffin in the morning with wheat toast and all-fruit preserves spread on top. Skip the mayonnaise and croissant for your turkey sandwich at lunch and replace it with two slices of hearty whole grain bread with mustard. When snack time hits, opt for celery without the peanut butter in the crevice, and add protein to the meal by drinking a cool glass of fat-free milk.

You can enjoy the delicious food at the wedding without guilt because you planned ahead. Using a food diary helps some individuals while others like to plan their food budget in their head. Think of the upcoming week. Decide when you might be eating rich desserts, high calorie foods, or fatty foods. From there plan ahead and you will have an easier time deciding what to order Monday for lunch… the grilled chicken fresh green salad or the big fat burger and fries!

5.

RATING THE DIETS

Let us rate the diets popular today. Americans spend billions of dollars each year only to gain the weight back. Wouldn't it be nice to be in a successful weight loss program? Here is an analysis of the different diet plans that are commonly available.

Slim Fast™ – This one is simple, inexpensive and requires no thinking. All you have to do is drink one shake for breakfast and lunch, and then eat a regular-sized healthy dinner. The drinks are full of healthy vitamins and minerals fulfilling your Recommended Daily Allowance.

Your wallet: 90 cents per serving.

Analysis: What happens if your "normal" dinner turns out to be a king's feast? This is because you have deprived yourself of chewing wholesome food all day. Chewing is extremely important for people to feel gratification. Fiber is necessary for intestinal health. Ultra Slim-Fast™ has five grams of fiber per serving. If you rely on the Ultra Slim Fast™ shakes, you may receive enough fiber for the day. It is not a diet you can use to change lifestyle habits.

Grade: D

Weight Watchers™ —It is easy to learn, affordable, healthy, targets all aspects of weight loss, and most importantly, is good for life.

Your wallet: $100

Analysis: This plan requires tracking, time, and effort. You will track your intake through "points". Different foods have different point values. This makes it easier to calculate how much you ate in a day as compared to counting calories.

Grade: A

Dr. Atkins™ - A diet consisting of protein with minimal carbohydrate.

Your wallet: $7.99

Analysis: This diet is not suitable for life. A lot of people do it until they lose the weight. But what are you to do once the weight is gone? You will gain weight back because you did not learn how to eat healthy. If you choose to follow this plan you will have the following risks: cardiovascular disease, cancer, hypertension, diverticulitis, diverticulosis, among other problems.

Grade: F

Richard Simmons™ – His plans teach you healthy eating for life. Some examples of plans are Deal a Meal™ and

Blast Off the Pounds™. These plans involve tracking your eating.

Your wallet: $39.95

Analysis: There isn't a health professional available to guide you. It is wise to have a counselor to ensure you do everything correctly. The plan is colorful, creative and fun.

Grade: A-

The Zone™ – Forty percent of your calories come from carbohydrate, thirty percent is from protein and thirty percent from fat. It claims to balance your hormone levels, boost metabolism, and raise your energy level.

Your wallet: $25 for the book, $1470 includes meals for 6-weeks (available only in a few major cities).

Analysis: Nutrition experts recommend having fifty to sixty percent carbohydrate and twenty percent from protein. Anytime you eat, you do boost the metabolism, whether you eat protein are carbohydrates. Too much protein is harmful for the health of your kidney.

Grade: C

Diabetic Exchange System™ – It is the basis for many legit diets like Weight Watchers™, Richard Simmons™, and diets created by Registered Dietitians. You consume three equally sized meals plus one to two snacks.

Your wallet: $40 - $65 per visit with dietitian

Analysis: The plan requires effort and time just as any worthwhile life change does. The benefits outweigh this one small negative. The plan is not only for diabetics. It is suitable for the healthiest Olympic non-diabetic athlete.

Grade: A-

USDA Food Guide Pyramid™ – It is shaped in a triangular pyramid for easy-to-remember visualization. The pyramid is split into six food groups. You eat more of the food group at the bottom of the pyramid occupying the most space.

Your wallet: $0, taught at public schools and listed on your grocery boxes (cereal).

Analysis: The top of the pyramid (sweets and fats) indicates, "Use sparingly", which is difficult to quantify. Make sure you measure all servings. The plan is very healthy when you follow it correctly.

Grade: A

No diet is good if it does not teach you how to eat for a lifetime. You should be able to enjoy your favorite food in moderation while continuing to lose weight. Eating food is a blessing that we should not abuse, but appreciate!

6.

EATING LIGHT ON THE BORDER

One of the most popular ethnic foods is Mexican. Mexican food has a bad rap for being fattening. This is not always so. Just as with any other type of food, if you know what to look for in terms of lean options, you most definitely can eat healthy Mexican dishes.

One of the first things you should do at a Mexican restaurant is skip the basket of chips. Maybe have one or two at the most. Save room for your stomach to have the "good stuff". This will be well worth giving up the chips. Is it too difficult for you to sit there and watch everyone eat chips? Put lots and lots of salsa on your plate and take only one or two chips to make it last. The salsa is fat free and low in calories.

If you must drink, I recommend going for a light Mexican beer. Have a lemon or lime wedge to jazz it up a bit more. Then you won't feel left out when your companions order the festive Margaritas. Twelve ounces of light beer is about 200 calories less than a margarita.

When looking at the menu, pass on the crispy fried chimichangas. Don't be fooled by the taco salad and think it's healthy! The bowl it is served in makes it similar to the chimichanga, just with more lettuce and less meat! If you want the taco salad, eat everything but the bowl and go easy on the cheese and sour cream. The deluxe nachos are another menu item that is a diet stopper. It's not really the style of cooking that makes Mexican food fattening, it is more so the ingredients and the toppings.

There are three ingredients to be leery of when eating Mexican. They include: cheese, sour cream, and guacamole. Ask for these items to be left off of your entrée, or order them on the side. Another idea is to choose just one and leave the other two off. I recommend going with the guacamole for its healthy content of monounsaturated fat. Do this especially if you have high cholesterol. The cheese is also a good choice for your one indulgence. Be sure to limit yourself though. Cheese is rich with calcium and Vitamin D. Especially if you are a woman who wants strong bones and to prevent osteoporosis. Here are some healthy Mexican choices that you can have for your diet:

Fajitas – Ask for your fajitas to be made with minimal oil. This will make them even healthier. The corn tortillas have more fiber and less fat as compared to the flour tortillas.

Burritos – They come in all different sizes from normal to gigantic! I've seen Mexican restaurants advertise their burritos as being "as big as your head". If it's beyond normal size be sure to split it in half and enjoy it today and tomorrow. You can also share it with your companion.

Tacos – Opt for the soft shell tacos. The hard shells are just like eating a bunch of corn chips. Try a fish taco if you haven't already. This Baja Mexican rendition is very healthy because they are made with broiled flaky fish. The sauce makes it really tasty!

Chicken fajita salad – This is usually made with your health in mind. Sometimes they are served in the big taco shell bowl. If so, ask to have it served without it. The chicken fajita salad is usually made with stir-fried chicken and vegetables and a bit of cheese. Ask for the cheese on the side so you can limit yourself to two spoonfuls. Use salsa as a dressing and you have a very healthy delight!

Most Mexican food is served with beans and rice. Both of these side items are extremely healthy. If you are trying to lose weight, eat one or the other. Beans are full of fiber, vitamins and minerals.

Start your meal with a salad. Ask for no dressing. Use the salsa on the table for a low calorie fat-free dressing. If the restaurant has fat-free ranch, you can mix that with some salsa. This makes a creamy spicy dressing.

Skip dessert. If you must have something sweet, opt for a cup of coffee with a little sweetener and skim milk. The best part is feeling satisfied after a Mexican meal. That's what keeps us coming back for more!

7.

JEALOUSY CAN WORK FOR YOU

Jealousy is one of the worst feelings a person can have. Body image is one of the things that people get jealous about. Your body image is related to what you eat.

We make looking good such an important part of our lives. Unfortunately people ridicule fit and healthy people. Why? Most of the time it is because they are jealous. They are uncomfortable with themselves and wish they had what those fit people have.

Has anyone ever been jealous of you? Your hard work and dedication to fitness and nutrition may aggravate the people you know. In this case you can keep a sense of modesty and compassion towards those that are jealous of you.

Have you ever made fun of someone just because they were eating something healthy? We all have. Many times that comment stems from envy and feelings of inadequacy. We should not judge others because what really matters is our own health.

You can redirect your feelings of jealousy to make it work positively for you. You may be jealous when you see another person's fit body. Maybe you cannot stand that person's ability to control what he/she eats. You need to take all of that envious energy and channel it directly to making yourself someone *you want to be.*

Run a mile to release your negative energy. Turn into the fitness enthusiast you desire to be. Next time you want to skip your workout, think about that fit person you are jealous of. This pain will motivate you to workout. You will have a sense of accomplishment and you'll do it over and over again. Change yourself instead of harming others.

Jealousy is a human emotion we all feel. It is nothing to be ashamed of. It is far better to admit to it and positively act upon it. Realize your downfalls and change them. Soon *you* will be the source of others' envy!

8.

BEANS, BEANS, OH MAGICAL FRUIT

I'll never forget my first day of history class. The professor wanted the forty-student class to become more acquainted. He asked each one of us to stand up and introduce ourselves. He wanted us to tell everyone our favorite food. I stood up and announced, "I love legumes!" I have delighted in the taste of legumes (beans) long before I became an R.D. Legumes are different than most other plants we eat. In particular, legumes provide a good amount of protein. This is because legumes grow in soil and trap nitrogen from the air. Nitrogen is an element contained in protein.

Beans are the "magical fruit" because of their rich nutrient content. These low-fat treats are a wonderful source of vitamins and minerals. This includes calcium; folate, iron, magnesium, niacin, potassium, riboflavin, thiamin, vitamin A, vitamin C and vitamin E. Beans also contain essential disease-fighting phytochemicals.

You can combine legumes with rice to obtain a complete protein. Protein is important for many bodily functions such as muscle development and hormone synthesis. Legumes are also rich in fiber. Fiber is extremely important for your health! It helps lower cholesterol, regulates blood sugar and prevents cancer and heart disease.

There are several ways to consume legumes. Have 1/8 cup of beans with your salad instead of croutons. You can also have them with soup, chili and casseroles. You can eat lots of Mexican inspired food! Mexican meals always come with beans! A bean burrito is an inexpensive choice that is tasty and healthy. Mash one cup of garbanzo beans with a teaspoon of lemon juice to make a Greek dish called hummus. Hummus makes a great dip for vegetables.

9.

GROW A MILK MUSTACHE

How incredibly fun it is to try to detect whom that famous star is hiding behind that big white milky mustache. After realizing who the star is, it is insightful to read the caption of how milk fits into that person's life. In all of the captions, you will notice that milk is portrayed as if it is a magical, powerful beverage.

Milk *is* a powerful beverage! For children, milk is a common drink to accompany two or three meals of the day. What happens to us as adults? It seems that somewhere around the age of thirteen we lose that very important drink in our life. Soda often takes the place of the creamy white beverage because of the taste. Or zero calorie water may replace milk for women who begin to watch their weight. Whatever the reason, there is no excuse for a lack of this important beverage in your everyday diet (unless of course you are allergic).

Speaking of milk allergies, many people say they are allergic yet they are not. Allergies to milk result in tragic situations such as hives, shock, and even death. Sometimes the enzymes that digest dairy products, called lactase, decrease with age. This results in poor digestion of milk products. This is called lactose intolerance. You can become lactose intolerant by refusing to drink milk for a sustained period. Intolerance to dairy products is reversible. If you are lactose intolerant try incorporating milk into your diet little by little. Try a little yogurt once a day for the first week. If you have a reaction, start with a smaller portion. Add a cup of milk to cereal in the morning for the next week. The third week you can try eating a slice of cheese pizza.

Milk is a rich source of calcium, Vitamin D, and riboflavin. It is vital for women to drink plenty of milk through the age of thirty. These years are the prime years for building strong bones. After age thirty, strong bone-building dramatically slows. This doesn't mean it is okay to stop drinking milk. You should drink milk throughout your life for optimal health. There is a high risk of osteoporosis for women who do not obtain enough calcium.

Does the taste of milk make your stomach turn? Here is one innovative and delicious way to drink milk:

Frothy White Delight
1 cup of milk (skim preferably)
4 teaspoons of sweetener of your choice (optional)
2 teaspoons of vanilla
14 large ice cubes

Place all ingredients in a blender and liquefy. Continue blending until it seems that all ice chunks have been chopped up.

Pour into a tall glass, top with a tablespoon of light whipped topping and a cherry if desired.

This white delight can also be made not so white by adding any one of the following:

chocolate syrup
teaspoon of instant coffee
strawberry puree
maraschino cherry juice

Get creative and make up your own mix-it-with-milk drink. There is no excuse for not drinking milk!

10.

GOOD FAT, BAD FAT

One of the most confusing segments of nutrition is the information regarding cholesterol. Cholesterol and fat are in your blood. They are key predictors of your future health. You can make changes nutritionally to make your blood full of the "good fat". This explanation will help you understand your next cholesterol test.

Good Fat - There *is* fat that is good! Consuming higher amounts of it is more beneficial than a low fat diet in general. Good fat increases the amount of "good cholesterol" HDL (high-density lipoprotein) in your blood. HDL decreases the amount of "bad cholesterol".

Bad Fat – This is fat that *increases* your risk for heart disease. It increases the LDL's (low-density lipoprotein) in your blood. You need to have low levels of these compared to the HDL's (the good guys).

Cholesterol – This fat is found in animal products including meat, eggs, fish, poultry, and dairy products. The liver makes cholesterol in animals as well as humans.

Total cholesterol – This is the total amount of your LDL's and HDL's. Under 200 mg/dl is desirable.

HDL – This is cholesterol that is composed more of protein than fat. HDL has important responsibilities in our blood. It's most important function is to draw the bad fat found in the blood back to the liver. The liver then eliminates the body of this fat. This is why the liver you eat is high in cholesterol. If you have a high count of HDL then you have lots of fat transporters removing bad fat from your blood. If you have low HDL, you will have a greater amount of bad fat flowing in your blood.

LDL – LDL is the opposite of HDL. LDL's are composed mostly of fat. You will have a greater risk of heart disease if your LDL's are high.

Triglyceride level – This is another measurement of fat circulating in your blood.

Trans fat – Margarine has trans fat. Although margarine is cholesterol free, the trans fat is not beneficial to blood levels. Trans fat tends to increase total cholesterol and LDL while decreasing HDL. The amount of bad fat in margarine is less than the amount of bad fat in butter.

How to achieve good cholesterol levels in the body (HDL level of 35 mg/dl or above):

- Exercise

- Eat foods high in monounsaturated fat like avocados, peanuts, natural peanut butter, peanut oil, olive oil and canola oil.

- Maintain a healthy weight

- Drink alcohol in moderation (1-2 drinks per day) Consult your doctor before using this as a preventative measure.

How to lower bad cholesterol:

- Having high HDL's.

- Eat polyunsaturated fats like vegetable oil, corn oil, soy oil, salmon and mackerel.

- Limit intake of saturated fats like animal fat, coconut oil and palm kernel oil.

- Eat soluble fiber like legumes, oat bran, and barley.

There is "Good Fat" and there is "Bad Fat". The next time you order your taco salad *with* guacamole, you will know that it only tastes great but it is beneficial too! It is better to eat the salad without the cheese or sour cream than it is to skip the guacamole.

11.

GRAZING

Grazing describes eating many small meals throughout the day. The number of meals can range from five to eight. Grazing is thought to be a healthy way to keep the metabolism running at a higher average. You give your metabolism a boost by eating a small meal every couple of hours. Think of it as adding fuel to a fire. When you need your campfire to burn stronger, you add more wood. This makes the wood burn faster.

How in the world could it be possible to eat eight times per day without gaining weight? These meals are what I call mini-meals. A trip to a Sunday all-you-can-eat brunch is not an example of a mini-meal. Gorging yourself is not a mini-meal. Even a combo meal at your favorite fast food restaurant is not a mini-meal. What is a mini-meal? See example diet below.

Diet for a healthy female (130 lbs)

8am – Wake up. 1 cup of oatmeal, 2 Tablespoons of dried fruit, ½ cup of skim milk with cinnamon and vanilla sprinkled on top of the oatmeal.

9am – Clean house.

10am - Spin up a fruit smoothie in the blender.

11am – Go for a 40-minute walk with husband.

12pm – Split a whole-wheat chicken burrito, low fat fish soft taco and ¼ cup of beans all smothered with salsa with husband. Drink a non-caloric beverage.

2pm – Stop by a Mexican restaurant. Eat one lean beef soft taco with lettuce and salsa. Drink water.

3pm – Golf nine holes at 3-par course with husband and friends.

5pm – Whole-wheat turkey sandwich with lettuce, tomato, and a side of fruit. Sip on water with lemon wedges.

6pm – Go shopping.

7pm – Sip on 4 ounces of white zinfandel mixed with 4 ounces of club soda and ice

8pm – More shopping.

9pm – Dine at an eclectic restaurant with husband. Drink water; split an order of scallops for appetizer, mixed greens sprinkled lightly with walnuts and pepper, six ounces of succulent pork loin, and a small lemony dessert.

10pm – Salsa dancing with husband.

This person thinks likes variety and enjoys eating. This is acceptable as long as the meals are healthy. You cannot eat cookies or fries for your mini-meals. You should eat whole grains, lean meat, veggies, fruit, etc.

I recommend grazing for anyone who enjoys eating frequently, hypoglycemic (low-blood sugar), and have the time to eat periodically. If you do not have the time to eat every two to three hours, pack a miniature boxed apple juice to sip at your desk or in meeting breaks. It all depends on your lifestyle. If you decide to try grazing, give yourself a couple weeks to get use to this new style. Your stomach will shrink and adjust to this new way of eating. Soon you will not be able to eat those large restaurant portions.

12.

THE TOP FAST FOOD CHOICES

Do you know which food items are wise choices at fast food restaurants? It is challenging enough to turn down the large fries. Use this quick guide to assist you next time you eat fast food. This is the healthiest option in regards to fat, calorie, vitamins, minerals, taste and price. You can add coffee, tea or diet soda as your beverage. You can also use mustard, catsup, barbeque sauce or pepper in moderation.

Arby's® – You can choose Roast Chicken Deluxe or Roast Turkey Deluxe. Order a garden salad as your side salad. Eat half of the salad and save the rest of it for later. Or you could share it with your dining partner.

Baskin-Robbins® – Try the "No Sugar Added Low-Fat Ice Cream". Thin Mint is a delicious flavor. Top it with chopped nuts and a sliced banana to make it a meal.

Blimpie® – This restaurant has several healthy options, as many sub shops do. You might like the Club Sub. Ask for whole wheat bread. Add many vegetables and a slice of cheese. You'll have a balanced meal in one sandwich!

Burger King® – Order the grilled chicken sandwich. Ask for the sauce on the side, and lightly spread it on. Have a side or garden salad with the yummy light Italian dressing to accompany the meal.

Carl's Jr.® – Try a tasty Chicken Salad To-Go™ with light Italian dressing. Nix the croutons and other toppings they give you. Sprinkle black pepper on the salad to give your salad a little kick.

Dairy Queen® - Order a single hamburger and a child size vanilla cone. No need to feel guilt. This meal keeps you right on track.

Del Taco® - Order the chicken taco salad without the sour cream. You can leave the guacamole because avocados are healthy. Add all the low calorie hot sauce you desire. Here's the difficult part. *Don't eat it the crispy fried shell!*

Domino's® – Order a 16-inch Hand Tossed Veggie Pizza, eat two slices and box the rest up for upcoming healthy meals. Accompany the pizza at home with a side salad.

Jack In The Box® – The Breakfast Jack® is an appealing sandwich. It's made from hamburger bun, a slice of cheese with ham and eggs.

KFC® – Try the Rotisserie Gold® three piece chicken. Eat it without the skin. It is quite filling. Order corn on the cob and baked beans as your sides.

Little Caesar's® Pizza – Choose the medium Round Cheese Pizza! Pizza!®. Add an individual size Tossed Salad with 1 Tablespoon of Fat-Free Italian dressing. Eat only one to two slices of pizza.

Long John Silver's® – The Flavorbaked™ Fish is flavorful and light. Accompany your meal with a side salad topped with fat free dressing, one serving of rice and one serving of green beans.

McDonald's® – Have the chef salad. Don't eat the bacon bits and croutons. Use the Lite Red Wine Vinaigrette. Add black pepper for flavor. A small glass of orange juice will accompany the meal nicely. Order a small cone of frozen yogurt for dessert.

Pizza Hut® – The salad bar can provide a filling meal that is healthy. If you do opt for the salad bar, beware of the not so healthy salad toppers. Pass on the thick crust pizza. Order the Thin N' Crispy® Pizza, cheese only or add as many veggies as you wish. Order a side salad with vinaigrette to eat before the pizza arrives. Salad will fill your stomach and take the place of eating too many pieces of pizza. Stop eating when full. Pizza is an easy food to forget that rule on.

Subway® - There are multitudes of healthy choices. Order the Veggie Delite ™. Start with a wheat bun then order the Subway ® sandwich artist to "load it up!" with veggies. Ask for vinegar, no oil and pepper on top. Order unsweetened ice tea spiked with a lemon wedge and you have yourself a very healthy and fulfilling meal!

Taco Bell®_- Choose the bean burrito! Ordering a soft chicken taco also is the best compliment.

TCBY® –Walk with a friend to the nearest "TCBY®" and order a kiddie cup of Regular Frozen Yogurt.

Wendy's® - Order a garden salad and a side order of chili to make a healthy taco salad. Pour the chili on top of the salad. Be careful not to burn your tongue as you try to gobble this scrumptious salad down.

Choose a recommended food each time you eat out. Be diligent to this rule and you may shed a couple of pounds easy!

13.

TOTAL COMMITMENT

The battle of weight loss, challenging yet attainable! When the goal is reached you will feel thankful that it was so challenging. There is no sense of accomplishment without the tough times. Total commitment is exactly what is required for weight loss. You need to devote your heart to a new nutrition and fitness lifestyle.

Many people start to lose weight and one month later give up. What is the difference between someone who loses weight and someone who doesn't? The people who lose weight do not have more time on their hands, they don't like to write in journals nor do they already eat healthy. They are all totally committed to the goal!

If someone said that your life depended upon improving your nutritional and fitness level, you most certainly would do it. And to be honest with you, your life *does* depend upon this.

Put 110% effort into reaching your goal. It won't come with any less effort. Don't follow a balanced nutritional plan some days and on other days take diet vacation days. That's not 110% effort. When the holiday season comes, don't compromise and gain weight. Continue exercising, continue budgeting your eating, and be healthy and happy!

How important is your nutritional and fitness goal? Is it worth passing up the traditional chip snack attack every night? Is it worth passing up one half-hour of television to take a refreshing walk? Is it worth fitting into your favorite pair of jeans? Is it worth being able to jog with your husband again? Is seeing your cholesterol drop worth it? *Yes, you* are worth it! Be committed!

14

DIFFERENT DIETS, DIFFERENT PEOPLE

People have different personalities. Diets that work well for some people do not work well for others. Here are some diets that are compatible to the different personality types:

> **Busy Bee** – You do not have time to follow a diet… playing around with lists of foods, counting calories and keeping track of exchanges. You have to make a change or else you won't live long enough to accomplish everything! You barely have time to exercise so you definitely don't have time to use a diet journal. The "Simple Diet" consists of five nutrition rules to live by. Spend two weeks practicing each rule until you've made it a habit. Here are the rules:
>
> - Eliminate refined sugar.
> - Eat plain vegetables for snacks, nothing else.
> - Drink only no calorie beverages.
> - Have a salad with every meal.
> - Make vegetables the largest portion of your lunch and dinner.
>
> **Lazy** – Are you too lazy to get up and change the channel when you can't find the remote? The "Journal Diet" consists of writing down absolutely everything you eat. You have to record everything. You even have to include the little bite you took of that cookie sitting on the

counter. The "Journal Diet" will help you because you will not want to expend the effort to write down everything. Therefore you will limit the amount of things you eat. Have a sponsor in your household police your journal. The sponsor must penalize you for each time you don't write a food down.

Balance Seeker –Your life is topsy-turvy just like your diet. You want to be a healthy person without strict rules. You need some organization. You are willing to compromise for a lifetime of health in exchange. Within this diet you will find the appropriate amount of food to eat to balance the body size healthiest for you. This amount of food will be determined by your basal metabolism. The "Calorie Diet" focuses on tracking the number of calories. You can find out how many calories you should eat by going to www.ediets.com.

Organized –You plan every detail of your life. You are the perfect fit for the "Diabetic Diet" from the American Dietetic Association and the American Diabetic Association. You will eat the same amount of food for all three meals. Planning meals ahead of time is not a problem since you are organized. A typical daily meal exchange consists of the following:

- 6 Starch Servings
- 3+ Vegetables Servings
- 2 Fruit Servings
- 5 Protein Servings

- 2 Milk Servings
- 3 Fat Servings

Visit www.eatright.org to find a dietitian that can help determine the correct meal exchange for you.

Budgeter – *You* like to call the shots. You are most happy when you are free to make your own choices. You like saving money for special occasions. You do not want to eat just because a diet plan says so. You want to be able to eat more on special occasions without guilt. The "Food Budget Diet" is similar to the "Diabetic Diet". However, you will have more freedom to determine when you eat and how much. You are given a weekly food allowance. You may use your allowance evenly throughout the day. You can budget your allowance for special times by eating light prior to the occasion.

Indulgence – Your personality does not allow you to give up things easily. As long as you could eat your favorite food every day, dieting would not seem so bad. Let's say you choose peanut butter for your "Favorite Food Diet". You can eat up to six tablespoons of peanut butter per day. You combine peanut butter with other food groups to equal your recommended allowance. Healthy eating plans can be developed around any indulgence.

Meatheads – You have an extreme personality. You are determined to get what you want. Are you convinced that you should eliminate your carbohydrates? You cannot do this while still being healthy. The "Moderate Carb Diet" will minimize your carbohydrate intake to five starch servings per day. This is low enough to lose weight but high enough to fight diseases and provide energy to be active.

15.

REALISTIC NUTRITION FOR BUSY BODIES

Some nutritionists are very extreme, opting for only organic forms of food, no refined sugar, or even prohibiting microwave use. These extreme measures might be more nutritious but are they realistic?

Here are the facts. We are busier than ever. Technology advancements have increased our ability to be more involved. Because we are on the go, our eating styles have changed dramatically in the last decade. We spend half of our food budget dining out. Thirty-four percent of it goes to fast food.

Choosing to follow a strict unrealistic diet will do one of two things. You will be hindered in your activity level requiring more time spent at home selecting and preparing foods. Or else you will become extremely frustrated after failing to be able to follow strict guidelines. You may become so frustrated that you abolish good nutrition. I have witnessed people do this and take a turn from being the ultimate health guru to an obese and unhappy person.

Instead, why not learn healthy tips to assist you in your "on-the-go" lifestyle? Fast food is not bad, but choosing fried food every time is. Try to eat fried food no more than one to two times per week. When you start limiting yourself you will enjoy the fried foods even more. The same rule should apply to your beverage selection and dessert. Choose these sugar-laden treats no more than once or twice a week!

What is a busy person to do then when dining out and looking for a non-fried side item? It is especially difficult at fast food restaurants to refrain from fried food. What I suggest is opting for the side salad. It can be difficult to pass up those crispy fries. Not only are they delicious but also they cost less! The restaurants tempt you by making the price low to choose the combo meal. Resist the urge and think long term instead of instantaneous gratification. You will spend less money on your health in the future by spending more money now going for the salad. You will be able to break your habit within a week or two.

I do not judge convenience, fast food, and eating out as bad. There *are* healthier options. However, busy people eat out because of convenience. Do this and you are making yourself even more efficient – eating healthy while accomplishing your goals!

16.

WHY EXERCISE?

Do you think that exercise doesn't play as much of a role in weight loss as dieting? Exercise is not just a tool for weight loss. There are other important benefits of this activity.

- Exercise is a mood booster. Have you ever noticed that when you exercise you feel better? This is because physical activity releases chemicals in the body that make you feel good. Take a jog if you feel stressed. You won't feel stressed when you come back!

- Exercise gives confidence. You will be proud for the time and effort you have put into working out. You are toned and look fantastically healthy!

- Chances of developing heart disease decrease when you exercise regularly. Your heart is a muscle. Exercise makes this muscle stronger. When your heart is stronger it is more efficient. It can pump more blood with every stroke. When your blood is pumping intensely during exercise it is clearing out your blood vessels. This prevents them from clogging as in a heart attack or stroke.

- Exercise prevents obesity. Excess pounds are caused by overeating and under-exercising. When you exercise you are burning calories instead of taking in. Keeping yourself from being obese is one health measure you can make that will decrease your risk in obtaining *several* other health problems. Cancer, heart disease, diabetes to name a few.

- Exercise improves circulation thereby giving you a nice healthy glow.

- Blood sugar regulation is prompted by exercise. Exercise will also help the diabetic reduce his/her weight. A ten percent decrease in weight can help improve diabetes conditions.

- Exercise increases the "good" fat within the body. The more HDL (the good fat) you have, the less your chance of heart disease.

- Women's risk of endometriosis is decreased with regular exercise.

- Your bones benefit! Ward off osteoporosis with weight-bearing exercise such as walking or swing dancing.

- Exercise increases the amount of hemoglobin in your blood. Hemoglobin is the oxygen carrier in the blood. This makes you less tired.

- Exercise revs up your metabolism. When you exercise you burn more calories, when you have more muscle, you burn a significantly larger amount of calories.

- Blood circulation increases with regular exercise. The chance of getting varicose veins decreases.

- Exercise makes the mind be more creative and alert.

- Exercising makes you more productive and efficient.

- Being active helps maintain your muscular strength, coordination and flexibility. These are helpful in preventing injuries later on in life.

- Your digestive system becomes more efficient.

- Cartilage in your body becomes thicker and more durable from regular exercise. This helps you withstand more impact with less injury.

So now you know why exercising is not just to lose weight. Exercise is for everyone and for several reasons. Be sure to check with your doctor before starting your exercise program.

17.

SALAD TOPPERS & DIET STOPPERS

What words do you think of when I say "salad"? Does the word "healthy" come to mind? You may be also thinking "disciplined dieter, green, low calorie, and nutritious." One of these doesn't always apply to salad. Which one is it?

Not all salads are "low-calorie". Some salads are higher in fat and calories than other tasty entrees on the menu. Here are the dos and don'ts of low-fat salad eating.

Do order a dressing on the side. Vinaigrette and Italian are good choices because you'll use less. They are not always lower in fat than their creamy counterparts. You should use *any* dressing sparingly regardless of whether it is low fat. You can use your fork to drizzle on the dressing.

Don't pour dressing on. Ordering a large salad instead of pizza is not necessarily being healthy, especially if you use too much salad dressing. ½ cup of salad dressing has more calories than two slices of satisfying pizza.

Do fill your salad with as many veggies as possible. How colorful can you make your salad? You will eat a wider spread of various nutrients if you select different kinds of vegetables.

Don't choose the fattening mixed salads like coleslaw, pasta salad, three-bean salad, Caesar, potato or ambrosia.

Do add flavor to your salad with calcium and Vitamin D rich foods. Try cottage cheese and use less dressing.

Don't add more than a spoonful of cheese. Cheese is high in saturated fat.

Do add a spoonful of healthy crunchy options such as nuts, sunflower seeds, or banana chips. Limit yourself to a spoonful since these are high calorie/high fat.

Don't choose the croutons, bacon bits, Chinese noodles, and fried onions.

Do add a bit of protein to your salad with turkey and ham slices, beans or chopped egg *if* you are making your salad your complete meal.

Don't add in large of amounts of protein unless you are making the salad your entire meal. Only use vegetables if the salad is accompanying your meal.

Do enjoy every bite of your salad. Savor the crunch and unique taste of each forkful.

Don't eat a salad for a meal if you're going to leave the table feeling unsatisfied. You are defeating the purpose if you eat again afterwards.

Salads can be a great way to eat a large quantity of tasty low calorie foods. Make sure you don't fool yourself into thinking you are eating less than you really are. If you follow the dos and don'ts, you are safe!

18.

NUTRITIONAL FACTS

Do you frequently read food labels? Reading a label and understanding it are two different processes. The label is titled "Nutritional Facts". This title is a requirement by the Food & Drug Administration (FDA) and the United States Department of Agriculture (USDA). The labels are required on all types of food except for foods that contribute few nutrients (coffee and spices), foods produced by small businesses and foods produced and sold in the same establishment. These are the terms you should become familiar with:

Serving Size – The label must have the serving size. This is a standard size determined by the FDA for consistency. This is based on serving sizes that people customarily consume. This allows you to compare products of the same type. The serving size may be less than what most people eat in a sitting. Do not assume that what you eat is one serving. For example, a small bag of chips is usually two servings. This means that you should eat half a bag of chips per meal.

Servings Per Container – The number of servings in the package of food. You can calculate this from the package size divided by the serving size. For example if the serving size is 8 oz and the package size is 16 oz, then the number of servings per container is two. Some people cheat themselves by looking at the calories and fat per serving.

They ignore the number of servings per package. So if there is two servings of chips at 150 calories each then the total is 300 calories. It is not the 150 calories that is printed on the label. That number is per serving.

Calories - The number of units of energy you are eating in one serving. If you expend as much energy during the day as the amount of calories you took in, your weight stays the same.

Calories from Fat - Examines the numeric value of calories that fat adds to the food.

Saturated Fat – The amount of saturated fat in grams. Remember this is the bad fat. Not more than 10% of your calories should come from saturated fat. There are nine calories per gram.

Cholesterol – The amount of cholesterol in milligrams. Consume less than 300 milligrams per day.

Sodium – The amount of sodium in milligrams. Consume 3 grams per day (3000 milligrams).

Total Carbohydrate – The amount of starch, sugar and fiber in grams. (4 calories/gram)

Dietary Fiber - The amount of dietary fiber in grams. Try to intake 20 grams of fiber per day.

Sugars – The amount of sugar in grams. Obtain only 10% of your calories from sugars. (4 calories/gram)

Protein – The amount of protein in grams. (4 calories/gram)

In addition, labels must present micronutrient content information for Vitamin A, Vitamin C, Iron and Calcium.

% Daily Value – Labels provide nutrient information in two ways. One is in quantities. The other is in percentages of daily values. The percent daily value column gives us an estimate of how the food contributes to our daily diet. Nutrient needs change depending on age, sex, height and weight and activity level. Therefore, the USDA proposed that the average American needs 2,000 calories per day. The % daily values on the label are calculated using a 2000-calorie diet.

Labels are only valuable to you if you know how to read them. If you understand this information you will be able to apply it and achieve healthful eating practices. The FDA has several programs to help educate the public. If you are craving more information on label reading, go to the following website:

http://vm.cfsan.fda.gov/label.html.

19.

CONVENIENT FOOD – GOOD OR BAD?

Are you hungry at work? Most work places have snack rooms stocked with nuts, buttery crackers, candy bars and cookies. Do you get hungry in a hotel room? Check out the well-stocked fridge in your room or the vending machine down the hall. Americans with a tight budget can opt for the 99-cent menu at most fast food restaurants. Food is available everywhere you go in America.

Is this a good thing or bad? Convenient food is beneficial for the active high school student who plays singles tennis. For the average person with a desk job, it is not. If the sedentary person is not cautious about snacking, convenient food can easily cause weight gain. Eating out of boredom, emotion, habit or addiction is easily possible through convenience foods.

How can we make food less convenient? Should we ban all fast food restaurants, refuse gas stations from looking like a mini-grocery store and prohibit donuts in the office? This would be impossible. There are two fundamental things you can do:

#1 – Munch on Healthy Foods - Think vegetables! Carrots, celery, red, yellow and green peppers, lettuce, radishes, turnips, eggplant, green beans and on and on. Change from chips, cookies and candy bars to fresh plain vegetables. Veggies are one of the best snacks. Sometimes vegetables do not provide the energy you need. You can also choose a snack that incorporates whole grains, healthy fat and protein. This includes granola bars or trail mix.

#2 – Increase Activities - If you do choose to continue to munch endlessly, you need to get a move on! You need to put all those extra calories to use by burning the extra energy. Most people do not have time or motivation to exercise a lot. Wouldn't it be much simpler to eat in moderation and exercise in moderation?

There was a group of people in the same enclosed environment. Various snack foods were readily available. These snacks were free. Two-thirds of these people were over their recommended body weight range. The overweight group chooses items such as these high sugar, high fat choices: vegetables with high fat dips, chips, buttery crackers, cheese, chocolate candies, cookies, pizza, and chips.

The healthy group's snacking habits varied. There were people within this group who snacked regularly and chose healthy whole foods such as fruits, vegetables, nuts and cheese. There were other people within this group that opted not to snack. The rest of this group had no continuous pattern of snacking. This group ate when they were hungry. These people listened to internal body cues for choices on when and what to eat.

People that snack smart tend to have more success with weight loss and weight maintenance. This can be difficult with the availability of convenience food. The key is to pay attention to your internal hunger cues rather than your environmental surroundings.

20.

CONFIDENCE IS PRICELESS

Body confidence is something many American women lack. The condition of low self-esteem is becoming more prevalent in men also. What does this have to do with nutrition and fitness? Body image applies to nutrition because eating disorders are a result of poor body image. A book I read, written by a registered dietitian, claims that 95 percent of all women have or have had some form of eating disorder!

Answer the following quiz question:

When you pass the fashion magazines at the check out line of a grocery store you feel:

    A. Jealous that I don't look like that.
    B. Depressed because I don't look like that
    C. Ashamed of my body compared to the cover model
    D. Fine. Who cares? I'm beautiful too!

If you answered D, you have graduated past this mindset. Reading this may give you insight on how to empathize with others. Most people would have answered A, B or C.

Comparing yourself to attractive people and feeling bad is a normal feeling to have once in a while. Just about everyone feels that way at some point in his/her life.

Notice the background of the attractive model. Pleasing background, I am sure. Whatever the case, it's a complimenting background to the person being photographed. Somewhere there's a background great for your unique look also!

The model is wearing expensive, trendy clothing. The clothes are perfectly tailored for that specific person. You probably didn't even know that the clothes on the side of the model that you can't see in the photograph, is gathered, pinned or ripped open for a perfect fit from the photographer's view.

Then there's the hair and makeup! She has professional make up and hair designers fussing over her for hours. Remember the last time you had your hair professionally done? How about the last makeover you treated yourself to at the beauty counter? Didn't you feel like a million bucks? You would look and feel pretty darn good too if a person fussed over every little detail on your face for an hour!

The picture the photographer took is perfect. The model has a perfect facial expression and a fabulous pose. That picture you see is not the one and only photo taken. What we don't see are the pictures where her face has an unattractive expression. For the cover photo they don't choose the picture where she is taken at an unflattering angle. You are looking at the best picture of five hundred taken.

Then they take the one picture and spend days touching it up. With a computer graphics editor we can take a few inches off her waistline, give her a fuller head of hair, erase those blemishes, smooth any wrinkles and brighten her eyes. I sincerely believe that each and every one of us could be a cover model after all that!

You have a unique beauty within yourself. Let that beauty shine. What is on the inside counts even more than the look on the outside. Smile and be confidant of who you are! Nothing is more gorgeous than a smiling face and everyone can have one of those!

21.

2 HYDROGEN ATOMS AND 1 OXYGEN ATOM

Consuming a plentiful amount of hydrogen and oxygen can help to improve your health and may even help in your weight loss efforts. What I am really trying to say is…drink WATER!!! And drink lots of it! I am sure you have heard these words countless times, but they speak the truth. Water is essential in maintaining proper health. Water is a part of every cell, tissue and organ in your body. It is also part of almost every function in the human body. Water helps to regulate your body temperature, transport nutrients, prevent constipation, cushion your joints and protect your body's organs and tissues.

Fifty to eighty percent of your body weight consists of water. A loss of 20 percent of body water can cause death and a loss of 10 percent can cause severe health problems. Adults can survive up to ten days without water in moderate weather and children can survive five days. In comparison, it is possible for a person to survive several weeks without food. Neither one of these practices are recommended. It is imperative to drink water frequently throughout the day and everyday. Your body does not store water efficiently, unless you are a camel.

You should not allow yourself to become thirsty. Your body is dehydrated when you do. I would recommend to everyone to sip on water throughout the entire day to keep your body from getting to this point.

Some people do not care for the taste of water. Sipping it all day can become boring. Try adding a slice of lemon, lime, orange or even a cucumber! Sparkling water is another option that is more filling due to the carbonation. Be careful of flavored sparkling waters. Flavored sparkling water may contain sugar. Check the label to see if there are any calories.

Water can assist in weight loss by helping to keep your stomach full. It also satisfies the need to have something in your mouth. Drinking water throughout the day will motivate you to make other healthy decisions. Weight management and exercise go together like peas and carrots. Being properly hydrated before, during and after your workouts will make exercise all the more enjoyable and beneficial.

22.

RENEWED MOTIVATION

Re-live the feeling from your childhood days when you bought your first pair of new tennis shoes. Maybe they were Velcro shoes, maybe they had zip pockets on the side, or maybe they even lit up when you stepped! You were very excited and couldn't wait to wear them!

Bring this sensation back and treat yourself to whatever it takes to make you exercise. It could be anything, a new Walkman, wristbands, outfit, tennis racket, or stopwatch. You could buy yourself a new bike to explore the back trails. For a real thrill, buy some roller blades to use by the beach or lake. Upgrade your skis to the latest design. Prepare for the new season by doing some weight training for your quadriceps, hamstrings and gluteus muscles. Buy a new set a golf clubs so you can improve your swing.

It doesn't have to be materialistic. Perhaps a membership to the prestigious fitness club that just opened. Some of the gyms today are becoming fun places to hang out. I've heard of spinning classes with karaoke! There are juice bars, salons, swimming pools and spas, volleyball courts and rock-climbing walls. You can join a local walking, running or biking club. Take an active vacation! Go white-water rafting in the Rockies, kayaking the glaciers in Alaska, walking and sightseeing at our nation's capital or mountain climbing in Maui.

Get started...go to the sports store, buy that club membership you want or make plans for your next great escape! Whatever it takes to renew your motivation.

23.

ANIMAL RIGHTS...HOW ABOUT HUMAN RIGHTS?

I love animals and I know so many of you do also. Even if you are not an animal lover, imagine you are. If you were an animal lover you would be.

Zoos have many positive attributes. For one, they educate us on animals. The zoo can be used as an example of nutritional diseases in living beings. Most orangutans, once brought into a zoo environment, will develop Type 2 Diabetes. This is because the zoo is a sedentary environment. Zoos are designed to make animals adapt easier to the environment. But it will never be the wide-open jungle they are use to.

We as more like monkeys than any other animal species. The Type 2 Diabetes is a direct result of decreased activity in the monkey. Does it sound cruel that this happens because of the environment that we put them in? Humans can contract Type 2 Diabetes from being inactive also. So why do we trap ourselves in our living room with a television? Are we really trapped? We can come and go anytime we please.

Do you work an extra eight hours on your day off? You should do something different that will benefit your physical health. You can mow and garden the yard. You can also give the house a spring cleaning. Do you spend half the day reading the Sunday paper? Try walking, biking or golfing instead.

We are similar to the monkeys in the zoo. Does the story about the monkeys irritate you? Use this anger to motivate yourself. Commit to breaking out of your comfort zone of sedentary life once a day. Like monkeys we are genetically made to be active. We have made our lives convenient with technology. Thus we are conveniently sedentary.

24.

FAT FREE CRAZE OF THE '90'S

Most people were fooled by the fat free craze of the '90's. The food manufacturers bombarded us with fat-free products. It was a sin to eat fat. A typical snack was three to four fat free cookies.

Many people don't realize that fat free products are packed with extra ingredients that still add calories. Fat is important. Fat is a tenderizer. It makes the cookies you bake soft and the perfect consistency. You may wonder how food manufacturers make fat free cookies so perfect. Packing extra sugar in the cookies makes up for the undesirable texture without any fat. Extra sugar means extra calories. Once you eat the cookie your body will store the extra calories as fat anyhow. Here are some advantages to having fat in your diet:

> **Satisfier** –Many times a fat free meal will leave a person asking, "How long until I eat again?" Tell me what makes more sense, eating an entire box of fat free cookies at 600 calories, or two small oatmeal raisin cookies at 110 calories? The satisfaction one receives from eating the fat in the oatmeal raisin cookies makes her stop at two. Otherwise she would continue eating the entire box of fat free cookies.

> **Good fat** – Studies show that people who eat a diet rich in the good fat (monounsaturated) have healthier cholesterol profiles than those who eat a diet very low in fat. Avocado, olives, and nuts are examples of the good fat!

Here are some advantages to having fat in your body:

Thermal – Fat keeps us warm. Having 0% body fat isn't desirable. You will be very cold if you have lower than desirable body fat!

Protector – Fat protects our vital organs from harm. Fat cushions us when we fall.

Americans *are* eating less fat. But we are becoming fatter! Americans have increased their caloric intake by 300 calories from the 1970's to the 1990's. That calculates to three-pounds every month!

Here is a basic guideline when eating fat free products. Eat in small quantities. Treat a fat free product as if it contains fat. For example, two small fat free cookies for dessert are part of a healthy diet.

Fat free is not the cure to bingeing, dieting, obesity or being overweight. Fat free products are designed to help you moderate the amount of fat you take in as a whole. Keeping the fat content in your diet around 30% is not the easiest change to make. Food manufacturers are helping you make this change with fat free products. If you need to lower the fat content to moderate levels choose fat free products in moderation. However, don't abuse them as so many people do.

25.

PROTEIN DIETS

Protein diets were hot in the seventies and early eighties, but disappeared when America went through its low-fat craze in the nineties. Protein diets typically are not low fat therefore they were not popular. Protein diets have once again become the means for weight loss. Many people have questions as to how this diet works. Is it good for you? Will you lose weight?

Yes, you will drop weight on this diet! However, a majority of what you lose is water weight. Carbohydrate is a water holding substance in the body. When you deplete your body of carbohydrate, you also dehydrate yourself. Therefore much of the weight loss is water.

The second reason you lose weight is because most people overeat carbohydrates. Consequently most commonly these are the foods with added fat (i.e. cookies, muffins, cake, croissants, etc.). Also, carbohydrates are readily available. When you pass by your secretary, she has candy on her desk. The vending machine is filled mostly with carbohydrate foods. So the real reason you lose weight when you eliminate carbohydrates is because you most likely overeat from this food group!

The bottom of the Food Guide Pyramid tells us that we should eat six to twelve servings of breads, grains, cereals, pastas, and potatoes per day. That is a lot! If you are an inactive forty-year-old female, twelve servings are too much. Try six. However, twelve servings are fine for a sixteen-year-old male playing high school basketball six nights a week. It depends on your activity level, age, gender and size. Six servings are not much. That huge morning bagel you pick up on the way to work counts as four servings of bread. Eat half of the bagel and save the other half for tomorrow.

Do you want to eliminate carbohydrates for the rest of your life? What are you going to do when your family goes out to your favorite Italian restaurant? Sit there and eat lettuce while they order ravioli, gnocchi, and lasagna? You might as well learn how to eat sensibly in any situation. It is possible to eat healthy at an Italian restaurant without putting on any weight. Share an order of angel hair pasta topped with marinara sauce and a light sprinkling of Parmesan cheese.

Protein diets do not teach you how to maintain your weight once you've reached your goal. You will gain your weight back if you go back to the way you were eating previously. A good diet should teach you new healthy habits to keep the weight off for life!

You should not do the protein diet for extended periods of time. This can do damage to the kidney. The kidney is an important organ in the metabolism of protein. Large amounts of protein make this organ work overtime.

Fiber is important to our intestinal tract. Eating a diet composed primarily of meat, cheeses, eggs and just a bit of carbohydrates does not supply enough fiber to the diet. Phytochemicals are disease-fighting chemicals found only in whole grains, fruits, and vegetables. Eating less of these will keep you from absorbing these disease-fighting friends into your body!

The foods eliminated in the protein diets are vital parts of our life in terms of health and pleasure. Anytime a diet plan totally eliminates a food group from your diet that is a sign that it is probably an unhealthy diet. In a healthy diet, all foods can be eaten in moderation. So instead of eliminating carbohydrates, just limit your intake to the recommended amount.

26.

"HONEY, IT'S YOUR TURN TO PICK."

One of my most favorite traditions I have is that my husband and I share our meals when we eat out. We started this healthy tradition several years ago.

The tradition began after eating a five-course meal at an expensive seafood restaurant. We both had our own choices that night. We ate every course of the meal, from appetizer to dessert. We had breakfast the next morning at another restaurant. I was not that hungry but I had an eight hour plane ride ahead – snacks only. I asked my husband if he wanted to split breakfast. He felt embarrassed because he thought it would be cheap. I assured him not to worry. We split a delicious egg skillet breakfast and walked away from the table satisfied and not overwhelmed with fullness.

Who would have ever thought that this was the beginning of a great tradition and a beautiful relationship? We still continue to share every meal that we eat out. We do this primarily for the health benefit. Are you the type that eats everything on your plate no matter how full you are? Both my husband and I are. Now we eat fifty percent less calories.

Have you ever shared a meal with your significant other? You probably walked away from the table feeling satisfied and not too full. Sometimes restaurants charge for the extra plate but usually include an extra starch and vegetable.

You may be thinking that it will be too difficult to choose a dinner you both like. My husband and I have a system that works quite well. We take turns choosing what we are going to eat each time we eat out. When I say, "honey, it's your turn to pick," my husband reads the menu and chooses three dishes that he likes. From those three, I choose the one that we order.

You and your significant other will introduce each other to foods that you normally would not choose. There *will* be times that you will not have enough food by splitting. You can try having a salad or appetizer before the meal and a dessert after. Give it a try the next time you go out for dinner. It's a great way to have fun losing weight!

27.

HOW SCIENTISTS ARE HELPING YOU EAT

Does the acronym GMO mean anything to you? Some people are receiving misinformation about GMO and are frightened by it. Other people are unaffected by this term, not scared at all. Some people don't even know what GMO stands for. GMO stands for "genetically modified organisms". Sound scary? It's nothing to be worried about.

The world's population is growing faster and more land is being used for urban communities. We have new housing developments, shopping malls, golf courses, parks and industrial centers. Have you ever stopped to think about what this land was used for before this growth? Most of the land was used for agriculture. California is a great example. This state is the agriculture capital of the nation. It also has one of the highest growing populations. Economists have predicted that California will lose twenty-five percent of agricultural land this century. That is enough to feed more than one third world country. Anaheim, home of the 2002 World Series Champion Angels, used to be orange groves in the 1950's. Now Anaheim is the second largest city in metropolitan L.A.

As you can see, we need a way to produce more food with less space. GMO is used to make crops grow and ripen faster. Plants are more resistant to bugs and deadly microorganisms. Best of all, our food is more plentiful in nutrients. Scientists have done this through altering the genes of food.

Do you think you have ever eaten a GMO food? Sure you have. Much of the produce you buy is GMO. Notice how big and red strawberries are. These strawberries are mammoth compared to what we were use to. More than likely, these strawberries have been genetically modified.

There is *nothing* harmful about them. These berries are beneficial to your health just as any other fruit and vegetable is. The fact that these strawberries are available for all seasons is the result of GMO. Without GMO, the crop yield may have been much smaller leading to absolutely *no* berries in your market.

GMO's help change produce to make them delicious, strong, juicy, succulent, and more resistant to bad weather and pests. So what is the big scare? GMO's are a new technique and "new" often scares people. In anything, there is always a resistance to change. It is not worth your time to worry. The Food and Drug Administration would not approve the GMO process if it were bad for your health. GMO's are one solution to a very complex problem. Without GMO's there are not enough fruits and vegetables to go around.

28.

CHINESE CUISINE

Chinese cuisine is touted as one of the healthiest styles of food. The evidence is in health statistics. The Chinese obesity rate is extremely low even though they eat more calories than Americans! Only 0.004 percent of men die of heart disease in China. The average Americans' cholesterol level is twice that of the Chinese. The Chinese eat half the fat and three times the amount of fiber as Americans.

Americans eat most of their Chinese food at restaurants. Recognizing which entrees are healthy can be confusing. Many of the entrees are heart healthy because of the stir-fry cooking style. Stir-frying uses a minimal amount of oil. Here are some great tips to remember next time you dine Chinese:

- **Arrival** – Chinese restaurants have an ambient atmosphere. Taking the time to enjoy this aspect of dining increases your overall satiety.

- **Beverages** – Try having some herbal hot tea with lemon. Sip on your tea throughout the meal. This will help slow your eating pace.

- **Appetizers** - Start with a bowl of soup such as Egg Drop Soup, Wonton Soup or Hot and Sour Soup.

- **Entrees** – Try anything with the words "Chow Mein". This is a healthy stir-fry of chicken, shrimp, beef or pork with vegetables, served with soft noodles.

- Or you can try Lo Mein. It's a similar dish with a different twist.

- Stir-fried beef, pork or chicken with black bean or garlic sauce is another option with lots of flavor.

- If you like omelets, try the Egg Foo Yung. It is similar to an omelet with vegetables, and your choice of shrimp, chicken, beef or pork.

- Chinese Vegetables with Shrimp, Beef, Chicken, Pork or Tofu.

Ignore foods on the menu that include: egg rolls, fried rice, and fried crispy noodles. Refrain from munching on the complimentary fried noodles brought to the table before your meal.

While you're out to eat, notice what your meal consists of. Think of the reasons for the incidence of heart disease being so much lower in China than in America. We've already discussed that they cook with less fat and eat more fiber. But there's one big difference. The larger portion of their meal is vegetables and grains. This is ideal. Americans typically eat the reverse. The largest portion being meat and little room left for veggies.

Learn from these observations and apply the same method to any meal. Go ahead and have that big juicy 12 oz. steak. Just split it with your friends so you have room for your vegetables!

29.

"IT IS ALL GOOD"

Do you know which foods are good and which ones are bad? It is "bad" to label food as being bad. People with eating disorders think this way.

Question: Is cheesecake good for you?
Answer: You bet it is!

Question: What about theater popcorn?
Answer: Yes, that too.

Question: Pork rinds?
Answer: Good.

Question: How about super duper combo meal?
Answer: Yes, of course and I am not telling you a lie.

Question: Chili cheese fries?
Answer: Absolutely *no* food is "bad" in moderation!

Have you read the latest nutrition news? One news article labeled a certain food "bad". Yet another article labeled the same exact food "good". Who's right? Who do you believe? It seems to be a matter of interpretation. I have one client who categorizes protein as healthy and believes that is the best way to stay lean. She is convinced that carbohydrates cause weight gain. This person will not eat pizza or spaghetti. I also have a friend who has a fear of meat and will eat nothing but carbohydrates. She loves vegetarian pizza and spaghetti! Exactly opposite of what the other weight obsessed person thinks. Both people are unhappy with their bodies and have not yet found what eating in moderation means.

We should all know that *all foods are good*. We have been misguided. This is bothersome. It hinders a person's ability to have a totally healthy attitude toward food. Having a healthy food attitude is essential to being a happy person with a positive body image.

On Friday mornings my dad always treated my family to a homemade pancake breakfast. I would never ever have butter on my pancakes. I did use lots and lots of "fat-free" syrup though! Not too mention, extra pancakes. I saved about 40 calories by not having butter. I added about 300 calories of syrup and pancakes to make up for what I was missing.

Compare the before and after:

Typical 1992 breakfast:	10 years later:
5 – 6" pancakes 1/3-cup light maple syrup Butter	2 – 6" pancakes 1-teaspoon butter 1/8 cup maple syrup
650 calories	350 calories

That was the mentality of many in the 1990's. We were convinced that anything fat-free was safe. Contrary to belief, fat-free is not calorie free!

My fear of butter is an example of what happens when someone believes a food is "bad." By eliminating a food from my diet, I was no longer satisfied. Therefore it was counter productive. The bottom line is don't eliminate anything from your diet.

30.

THE POWER OF MEDITATION

As you change some of your life habits to healthier ones, there is one aspect of health that should not be forgotten. This is the power of your inner spirit. Everyone has a spirit; it is just a matter of finding it. Finding your inner spirit means finding peace and solitude within yourself. Discovering your inner spirit will help you to reach your health goals.

When challenged with difficult situations, you can use your spirit for support instead of eating. Some people eat when they are stressed. You can control stress with your spirit *but not by eating.*

You may be wondering, "How do I find this inner spirit?" It takes a lot of discipline. You need to set aside some time each day to relax. Let your mind go blank. It is okay if you cannot clear your mind completely. Perhaps the thoughts remaining in your mind are troublesome. Acknowledge these thoughts. Set them aside. You are beginning meditation.

Find a place where there are no distractions. Open the windows and allow the peaceful sounds of nature to fill the room. If it is cold outside, you can use a nature tape or CD. Light a candle if you desire. The morning is an exceptional time to meditate. There is less commotion and it sets the mood for the day.

You can incorporate breakfast if you feel hungry. Choose something light with carbohydrate. An English muffin or a handful of raisins will help your mind stay focused.

You can also include fitness into your meditation. Try taking a walk or doing yoga. Another great way to relax is by taking a bath. You can use a lavender oil, salt or bubble bath. Surround the tub with candles.

After you have cleared you mind, it is time to meditate. Meditation can be prayer or brainstorming. Writing in a journal is another style of meditation. You can read a self-help book with inspiring-stories. Read each passage and think how to apply it. Let it help you become a better person.

How should you soul search? Here are some excellent things to think about during your meditation:

- Your strengths and weaknesses in healthy eating.

- Challenging your workouts.

- The person you admire for his or her healthy lifestyle. How can you be similar?

- The place where you feel accepted for who you are.

Choose a meditation style that suits you. Realize that it takes discipline and consistency. It is important to allow yourself stress free time every day. Frequently putting your mind at ease will eliminate stress. Soon you'll smile and say, "I am healthy - spiritually, mentally and physically."

31.

ASSERTIVE DINING

Being assertive in life can bring you an abundance of success. Ponder for a moment what being assertive means to you. You may think assertiveness is in the work place or in relationships. Have you ever considered being assertive in the realm of health and nutrition? It could be very beneficial.

My client, Dee Ann was dining at a popular pizza place. She ordered a small pizza and a side salad. Since Dee Ann is weight-conscious she budgets what she eats. She ordered the salad with *fat-free dressing on the side*. Dee Ann knows pizza is a high calorie food so she wants to balance her meal accordingly. The server brought the salad but the dressing was not on the side.

"Oh well, at least it is fat-free…or is it?" She thought. She looked closer and realized it was not fat-free. This is not what she ordered. Dee Ann continued the rest of her meal without saying a word to the server. She felt frustrated because she was *trying* to limit her calories.

Dee Ann could have prevented her frustrations. She should have sent the salad back since the dressing was not on the side. Don't be afraid to command perfection when you dine out. Ask questions about what you order. Many servers think regular Italian dressing is low fat. Italian dressing is not always low fat! You may also want to know how your food is prepared. Remember every calorie counts. If you are served regular soda instead of diet then send it back.

What about when you are dining in the company of others? You need to be assertive in this situation also. Know in your mind what you can afford to eat and consume accordingly. Ignore the comments about what you eat. Don't let friends or family persuade you into eating more when you have had your fill. Be assertive and stick to your original plan while politely letting the comments pass without verbal retaliation. And remember, as little contact with negative people as possible is most beneficial to the new healthy you!

Being assertive does not mean you have to be pushy. That would be aggressive. It is having a goal and striving to accomplish it. As you already are aware, being assertive on the job, at school, in sports and clubs will take you far and in the direction you choose to go. Nutrition and fitness combined with an assertive attitude will help you achieve more results. Assertiveness is, essentially, priceless!

32.

BALANCING YOUR LIFE

What makes up whom you are? Have you ever thought about that? This is an interesting thought and a provoking question. Some believe there are three parts to every human. This is similar to fruit. There is the skin, the juicy inside and finally, the seed. All three parts are different however they are all important to making up the fruit as a whole.

The physical self is comparable to the fruit skin. It is the outer covering that everyone sees. Does a bruised rotting fruit sound appealing to you? Probably not, nor do you appeal to yourself when you fail to maintain your health, hygiene and outer appearance. Washing your hands often, eating a well-balanced diet, exercising several times a week and looking clean are important factors to your self-perception.

The inner self is analogous to the flesh of the fruit. The inner part of the fruit is full of nutrients to make us healthy. Our inner self-functions like this also. We have a brain to think with. We can nurture it through challenging activities. The inner self goes far beyond traditional education's boundaries. The inner self includes music, dance, art, and writing. Its possibilities are endless. You can bring so much good to the world if used properly. It is important to make you inner self-healthy just as you make your physical self-healthy. Learn, challenge and expand your mind. You must concentrate on your inner self for optimal health.

The spiritual self is like the seed of the fruit. This is the most difficult of all three parts to explain. It is energy, excitement, emotion, peace, self-actualization and satisfaction. There are several activities to develop the spirit. Find it through meditation, mantra, yoga, reading or church. Choose what is best for you. You are you because of your spirit. Take time to nourish and develop this part of yourself. Spend at least ten minutes a day in deep thought and relaxation. All aspects of your life will come together. Problems will be manageable. For example, losing weight will be less difficult. With your spirit, you have the capacity for change. You have the power to brighten another person's day. Whether or not you use this power is up to you.

Being healthy does not only involve exercising and eating a healthy diet. True health comes from developing all three parts of the self to make the whole complete. One of my former clients worked as an influential contractor to a prestigious company. She spent most of her time and energy on the inner part of herself. As a result, she was obese and felt distressed often. She didn't care to eat healthy or exercise. Nor did she nourish the spiritual self. Once she realized these weaknesses, she was able to regain control. Since then she has become more efficient at her professional life as well as a healthier individual.

33.

AN EXERCISER'S BEST FRIEND

Having a dog can be a great way to stay active. One of the great aspects of having a dog is that you need to walk them. I walk my dog every morning, afternoon and evening. These walks are for short distances, usually just 15 minutes. But if you do this three times a day, it adds up to 45 minutes of exercise. On weekends you can go for longer walks. Perhaps you are having a difficult time motivating yourself to exercise. When you have a dog, you are forcing yourself to be active. You will also be helping your pet stay healthy.

Studies have demonstrated that pets are healthy for your mental status. Pets make you smile and laugh. They also keep you from feeling lonely. A recent poll in "Spirit" magazine claims that 64 percent of people talk to their pets first before they speak to their spouse!

If you have desired to own a pet and likewise you need a reason to exercise, there couldn't be a better time to adopt a best friend. Be sure to treat your pet right by giving him lots of love, attention and WALKS!

34.

"ENJOY" FOODS FOR YOUR HEALTH

Studies prove that people who enjoy the food they eat absorb nutrients better. Our physical health collaborates with our mental well-being. Many countries promote this concept as a guideline to live by. Other countries advise people to eat foods they consider "delicious".

A group of Thai and Swedish researchers examined this interesting concept. They took two groups of women; one group was from Thailand while the other group was from Sweden. The women were all served a popular Thai dish of rice and vegetables spiced with chili sauce, fish sauce, and coconut cream. Remarkably, the Thai women absorbed more iron from the dish than the Swedish women did. The Swede's labeled the dish as "too spicy". The researchers processed the identical dish in a blender and served it to the same women. All of the women ate the disgusting looking mush. The iron absorption rate fell dramatically by 70 percent!

All too often we eat on the go, in the car or at the desk while working. Try sitting at the table each time you eat. Take the time to taste each bite of food. This will signal the body to absorb nutrients more efficiently! This will also keep you from eating too much.

Eat foods that are appetizing to you. I am not advocating eating burger and fries every meal if that tastes best to you. You should still eat healthy foods. You need to find a fun and appetizing way to eat them.

Don't always follow a diet plan word-for-word. Change it around to suit your appetite. By making it appealing to your body you will end up with healthier results.

35.

SEVEN WAYS TO EAT A TATER

Potatoes are a carbohydrate-rich food. We tend to like them prepared with added fat. Naturally, they are fat-free and cholesterol-free. Potatoes are a wonderful source of vitamin C and potassium. They are also a good source of vitamin B6 and dietary fiber. The most common way we eat potatoes are French fries. Unfortunately French fries are fattening. In fact, most of the ways we eat potatoes are not for everyday consumption. Don't be discouraged. Just one potato with the added toppings is all you need for a delicious and quick meal! Here are seven ways to keep your potatoes nutritious!

> **California Style** – top your baked potato with fresh cooked veggies such as broccoli, cauliflower, carrots and onion. Add imitation butter, a little salt and pepper to taste.

> **Wisconsin Cheese Style** – bake a potato and while it is still hot sprinkle a couple tablespoons of low-fat cheddar cheese on top.

> **Texan Style** – smother your potato with chili. Make sure that your chili is prepared with some type of lean meat, poultry or tofu along with delicious beans.

American Style – You won't have to miss eating French fries. Bake a potato and make four long slices while it is still warm. You can chop each slice in half if you wish. Spray with cooking spray or light margarine spray. Lightly salt the wedges. Add ketchup in a mound on the side and dip away!

Southwestern Style – spice up the potato by adding salsa. Top with fat-free sour cream. Ole!

Western Breakfast Style – chop a warm baked potato into one-inch cubes. Cook diced onions over medium-high heat in a skillet filled with enough water to cover the onions. (Add more water if the pan becomes dry.) Add four egg whites or ½ cup of egg substitute and 2 tablespoons of skim milk. After the eggs are somewhat set, immediately take the skillet off the heat and add the potatoes. Season with salt and pepper.

Chinese Style – stir-fry ½ cup of frozen Oriental-mix veggies in 2 teaspoons of canola oil. After a couple of minutes, remove from heat and top split baked potato. Add a few splashes of soy sauce.

Enjoy these fabulous creations! You can use different types of potatoes. Sweet potatoes add more Vitamin A. You can make your own healthy combinations.

36.

A GUIDE TO HEALTHY ETHNIC EATING

If it weren't for my knowledge of low-fat, low-calorie ethnic foods, I probably would not have control of my weight. Both my husband and I love Mexican food. One-third of our meals are Mexican! Many people perceive Mexican food as fattening and some of it can be. However there are healthy ways you can continue to enjoy your favorite ethnic foods.

Mexican - What happens when you first sit down at a Mexican restaurant? The server brings a basket of tortilla chips and salsa. Most people fill up on the chips *and* eat the meal too! Treat yourself to only a few chips or none at all. Move the chips out of your reach to avoid your temptations. The salsa is very low fat and low-calorie because it is really just a bunch of vegetables minced together. You can also enjoy using salsa as a fat-free dressing on your salad. The fat lies in the heavy doses of cheese, sour cream, and deep-fried cooking. Choose the following Mexican foods infrequently:

Chimichanga
Nachos Grande
Taquitos
Taco Salad
Guacamole dip with taco chips
Crispy fried tacos or fried tortillas
Refried beans (in lard)
Tostados, quesadillas
Fried Ice Cream

These dishes are fried and covered or filled with cheese. One positive aspect is that Mexican food typically contains beans. Beans are a great source of B vitamins, protein and fiber. Eat these healthy dishes most often:

Veggie, fish or chicken fajitas
Bean, chicken or Vegetarian Burrito
Enchiladas or tamales
Refried beans (no lard)
Chicken or fish soft tacos

Mediterranean - This diet is one of the healthiest diets of all. The fat used in cooking is olive oil, which is a monounsaturated fat. These types of fats lower cholesterol. The protein source is most commonly fish. Fish contains essential omega 3 fatty acids. Eat the following foods moderately:

Moussaka (a layered eggplant, cheese and beef dish)
Spanakopita (a vegetarian egg, spinach, feta cheese dish)
Greek Salad with dressing already on the salad
Pastitsio – Greek Lasagna
Souvalaki – Lamb skewer

Choose a standard serving of these dishes if you are opting to eat light.

Avgolemono soup (a chicken, rice, vegetable soup)
Baba ganosh (similar to hummus)
Hummus
Tabouli
Tahini (sesame paste)
Yogurt and Cucumber Salad

Italian – Limit the amount of pasta you eat to one helping the size of your fist. Only have one slice of bread and regulate the amount of butter, margarine and olive oil. Drizzle salad dressing on with your fork instead of pouring it in huge amounts. The following entrees are higher in calories and fat:

> Eggplant, Chicken or Veal Parmigan
> Antipasto plates
> Buttered garlic bread
> Pasta with white sauces such as alfredo
> Italian sausage
> Cannoli

Better Italian food choices:

> Pasta with Marinara or red sauce
> Manicotti
> Chicken cacciatore
> Italian fruit ice

French – Mangez-vous Francais? Do you eat French? If you do, most likely you'll be eating the food of romance accompanied with a glass of wine. Only have two glasses. A dark red wine is most heart healthy. If you do not drink alcohol I am not recommending you start. Choose less of these when dining French:

> Cheese fondue
> Croissant (plain or chocolate filled)
> Escargots
> Sausage in brioche
> Salad Nicoise, with dressing

Hollandaise sauce
Napoleon (a puff pastry ice cream dessert)
Chicken cordon bleu

Instead go for these delicious delights:

Brioche
Salad Nicoise, with 1 Tablespoon of dressing drizzled on top
Bouillabaisse (a fish stew)
Ratatouille (an eggplant, zucchini, garlic vegetable side dish)
Profiterole with fruit (small puff pastry)

Japanese – a very popular fad in the new millennium is sushi. Dine in style however control yourself from having these choices to often:

Green tea ice cream
Tempura
Shabu shabu

Instead favor the following:

sashimi
Sushi, maki
Sushi, migiri

Eating ethnic food will add great excitement and diversity to your diet. It will also give you a combination of nutrients in new and different ways. The next time you are debating on what to eat you should try something new such as Argentine cuisine. Be adventurous and go for the unknown!

37.

DANCING MACHINE

Would you like a fun and exciting way to workout? Slide in a CD; turn on the radio, pop in a cassette, or get out the old records, whatever it takes to *dance*! Dancing is a fabulous workout. Time will fly because it is so much fun. It also enhances your mood. It's difficult not to smile while busting a move to your favorite song. There are numerous ways to dance. You choose what is right for you.

> **Ballet** – Ballet will help you become more graceful. Ballet helps tone your muscles. Ballet tones the lower half of your body such as the leg muscles (gastronomies, quadriceps, hamstrings, and inner thigh muscle). Ballet tones just above your leg - the gluteus maximum and minimums, and even down to the muscles in your feet from pointing and flexing. The upper body reaps benefits also. Abdominal muscles are toned from tightening to keep the body balanced as well as back muscles. With correct ballet arm movements, you can get rid of the fat on the back of your arm. Ballet also provides a cardio workout. Ballet improves flexibility. You will be able to touch your toes while keeping your legs straight. Lastly, ballet improves posture. It teaches you how to carry yourself with poise and confidence.

> **Hip-Hop** – How about an aerobic workout? Hip-hop makes you sweat. You can take a hip-hop class at a dance

studio to learn the moves. Many community colleges also offer hip-hop. You can watch a music video and mimic the steps. Some hip-hop dances incorporate many level changes. You'll switch from standing to squats and exercise leg muscles you typically don't use! Find that inner Michael or Janet Jackson in you and let it loose!

Country line dancing – You will be burning calories while "swinging your partner". You will make new friends when dancing with everyone in the circle. This dance is great for weight-bearing exercise. Your calves, hamstrings and quadriceps will benefit. You'll burn 8 calories per minute! This is comparable to a fast walking pace.

Ballroom dancing – You can learn ballroom dancing at a studio or college. Ballroom dancing includes salsa, tango, waltz, box step, rumba and mambo. The instructor will have you rotate partners so you dance with everyone. This helps you learn other dancers' style. You will burn 6 calories per minute doing this classic form of dance. This is comparable to a leisurely swim. Your leg muscles will benefit along with gluteus maximum, abdominal and oblique muscles (AKA love handle area).

Swing dancing – Get ready for some fabulous fun everyone can enjoy! This dance craze hit it big again in the late nineties. It is a fun and upbeat dance style derived from the forties. What a great feeling to be having fun while working out. You will burn six calories per minute with this form of dance. You'll work your leg muscles, gluteus, arms and abdominals.

Belly dancing – an up and coming trend in America. This form of dance originated from India. There are eleven forms in all which are particular to the different regions of India they stemmed from. Rajasthani is a dance, which consists of spins, backbends, protruding hip movements and balance. Try Filmi for the classical form of belly dancing. Filmi originated in Bombay. Bhangra is the most popular in India. It is well liked because of its catchy drumbeat. This form of dance is often performed at social celebrations. With belly dancing, you will be burning fat while toning your arms, abdominal, hips, thighs and your gluteus muscles.

Who cannot have fun dancing? It is one of the best ways to exercise! You can devote a few hours a week to dancing simply because it is a great way to make your heart beat. Step onto the dance floor and strike a pose!

38.

GOT CALCIUM

It is important to consume a lot of calcium, especially when you are younger. Most people do not realize that calcium affects your circulatory system. We all know that calcium is essential for strong bones. But it is also vital for your blood supply. Your bloodstream is first supplied with calcium. The remainder of the calcium strengthens your bones. Your blood relies on the calcium that has been stored in your bones if there is not enough calcium supplied in your diet. It is analogous to having overdraft protection on your checking account.

Your bloodstream needs calcium to regulate fluid in and out the blood cell. Rich sources of calcium include dairy products, shrimp, sardines, salmon, tofu and calcium fortified foods such as orange juice. Food is the best way to obtain nutrients. Calcium is no exception.

Another way to ensure you get enough calcium is through supplements. There is a wide variety of calcium supplements available. Choose the ones that contain calcium carbonate or calcium phosphate. Take two or three tablets per day with four to six hours between each tablet. Take each tablet within an hour before or after a meal. If you are using a liquid supplement, take it within an hour *before* a meal.

The body will only absorb about 500 milligrams of calcium at one time. If you are eating a high fiber meals (such as a fiber-rich cereal) opt to take your calcium supplement at another meal. Iron is also another nutrient that can inhibit calcium absorption. Take your calcium supplement at different times than your iron or multi supplement.

39.

A HEALTHY CHILD

Childhood is the time in a person's life when physical fitness, body image, and food habits are learned and attitudes are developed. It is a parent's responsibility to help instill healthy lifestyle habits into their children. As you read the following you'll see some of the most common questions parents ask dietitians.

Question: "My child hates vegetables! How do I get him to eat them?

Answer: Let's put ourselves in the child's shoes. Our taste buds change throughout the years. A child detects bitterness because his/her taste buds are sensitive. That explains why you once could not stand asparagus, but now think they are fine. You can mask the bitter taste of the vegetable by adding other flavors. For example, melt cheese on cooked broccoli. Spray a light margarine on cooked carrots. Fill the crevice of celery with peanut butter. Make green bean casserole. Cooked veggies are less bitter than raw veggies. The child will learn to appreciate these veggies and you eventually can try serving the vegetables solo as the child ages.

Question: "My child sees the veggies and refuses! Masking the flavor doesn't work! He's already tried them and won't try them again."

Answer: You could be sneaky and puree the vegetables and mix them in casserole dishes such as cheeseburger pie. Ask the child nicely to "please try the vegetables." Try to have the child eat one bite for each year the child is old. Maybe he/she idolizes a superhero that is big and strong. Explain to him/her that the superhero ate a lot of vegetables to become strong. Do not allow the child to have dessert if he/she won't abide. If the child asks for a treat later on…give the child the vegetables! If your child has a friend that likes vegetables, use this to your advantage at the dinner table. You could say to your son's friend, "These carrots are tasty, wouldn't you agree, Joey?"

Question: "My child doesn't like milk. Milk is so important for a growing child. What should I do?"

Answer: This could be a sign of milk intolerance. Intolerance is the lack of lactase enzymes to digest milk. Common side effects are indigestion, gas, diarrhea, etc. There are plenty of ways for children to receive the benefits of milk without drinking it. Some orange juices are fortified with calcium and so are some cereals and cereal bars. Supplements are another way to ensure children are receiving the nutrients. Most children love those little sweet vitamins.

Question: "How can I make my daughter be more active and watch less television?"

Answer: What type of television shows does she watch? This may give you an idea as to what kind of physical activity she would enjoy. Watching cartoons where characters are doing flips may interest her in gymnastics. Action cartoon characters also may be a clue to a child liking karate or tae-khan-do. If she likes to watch cartoons starring animals, maybe she would like nature hikes where you try to spot animals as you hike. If your child is watching sports on television, that's a clear sign of what she may be interested in.

Question: "Eating disorders seem to be so prevalent in teenagers. Is there anything I can do to prevent this from happening when my daughter grows up?"

Answer: If you want your daughter to have a positive body image, you need to be an excellent role model. Don't comment on how "fat your thighs are". Don't crash diet. Believe me; your child is able to tell when you are dieting. When you do diet, make sure you eat the same foods as the rest of the family, just moderate your portions. Model healthy eating habits you would like your child to follow. Be active and exercise consistently. Compliment your daughter not only on her physical beauty but also on her personality, intelligence, athletic ability, etc. The same goes for making comments about other people. Listen to your daughter if she starts making negative comments about her own physical appearance. Reassure her we all have those days and ask her if she thinks there is anything she could do to make herself feel better. When she is older, explain in detail the process behind making someone look good for the cover of a fashion magazine. The picture isn't real, just like a doll isn't real. And most importantly don't let her be influenced by the media. She is very vulnerable at this age.

40.

FOOD OBSESSION

Do you think about food all of the time? If you are dieting, these obsessive thoughts can make it even more difficult to persevere.

Food obsession can occur in many individuals, such as:

- Avid dieters who feel restricted from food

- Individuals with eating disorders

- Bingers

- Overweight or obese individuals

- Emotional eaters

- People who dream about food

- People who suffer from anxiety when they are in a food environment

If you have any of these problems, don't be embarrassed. Any problem is possible to overcome. Do not revolve your day around food. Food is simply energy, which allows you to perform. When you wake in the morning, meditate. Find strength and balance for yourself. Devote your day and evening to non-food related activities that occupy your mind. Since your mind is preoccupied, you won't have time to think about food.

Do you use getting together with friends as an excuse to overeat? Do a variety of activities. Don't go out to eat every time. Try doing physical activities such as dancing, bowling, and walking. When you do gather to eat, share low calorie versions of your high calorie favorites. Have a taste-test and let your friends rate the foods!

Do you obsessively think of numbers in terms of your weight, calories, fat grams, or food exchanges? The no diet-diet requires you to listen to your hunger. You can only eat when confronted with a hunger pang. Eat small one-portion meals. And only eat when you are sitting down. This will allow you to eat less and enjoy every bite. After a while you will not care about calories because you are able to eat by instinct.

41.

DEAR DIARY

Do you think a diary is only for deep dark secrets? Diaries can be used for food and fitness too. A journal can help act as an impartial listener.

People who are stressed mentally often allow their physical health to suffer along with their mental health. Some people eat food to relieve stress. When your body is stressed, treating it with proper nutrition is critical. Not eating healthy can cause a lack of vital vitamins, minerals and other nutrients. This causes the body to be highly susceptible to illnesses. It is just as bad to overeat from stress. People that are stressed chose comfort foods. These foods are more calories and fat. The weight gain can put more pressure on your heart physically and emotionally.

The journal is also a way to record your daily diet. Dr. Daniel Kirschenbaum, a psychologist at the Center for Behavioral Medicine in Chicago, compared two groups of dieters in an organized treatment program. The dieters who were faithful self-monitors and wrote down everything they ate, did not gain weight. Dieters, who skipped this part of their treatment program, gained an average of 10 pounds. Tracking what you eat every moment of the day makes you aware of how much you are taking in and reaffirms your commitment to losing weight. Try writing down everything you eat for a day. You will realize how much nibbling you are doing. All of this really adds up!

You can use a palm pilot or pocket PC to track your diet. The software program will allow you to check you fat, saturated fat, fiber, vitamin and mineral intake. The food database will automatically provide the calories, etc. for everything you eat. The program will also give you a running balance of how many calories you have consumed for the day. There are several other options for food tracking. You can buy a diet journal from your bookstore or you can use a service on the Internet. Do what works for you though so you can stay committed to it.

You should also journal your activities for each day. If you write down everything you do, you will have a sense of accomplishment. It will make you more aware of how much or how little you really exercise. A client told me he exercised four times a week, however after looking at two weeks of his journal; he averaged one exercise session per week. Track the amount of time you spend doing each activity. Also rate the level of energy for every activity. It's beneficial to choose activities with different energy levels.

I have assigned food journaling to several clients. This is a significant factor to the success of their weight control. You can keep a journal full of daily caloric intake, expenditure and feelings pertaining to food and exercise. If you do, it is extremely important to carry the journal wherever you go.

42.

SWEET AS SUGAR

In the 1990's, America went through a phase were we labeled fat as "bad". Food manufacturers began overwhelming us with low-fat and fat-free food items. Our mentality was, "If it's fat-free - we can eat as much of it as we want."

We were so wrong! Many of us thought we ate healthy because we ate low fat. The fact is, we were missing out on valuable nutrition.

Fat is important and necessary. Fat has significant functions in the body such as keeping us warm and offers us an excellent energy source. We need it only in moderate amounts and as Americans; we tend to abuse the moderate amount rule. Counting fat grams is important for weight control but what is even more important is counting calories. Sugar was used to replace fat. Sugar has fifteen calories per teaspoon, and no vitamins, minerals or protein. It might taste good but it's empty calories! Keep in mind that just because foods are fat-free *does not* mean they are calorie-free.

Be conscious of the sugar calories you consume. You know those little packets of sugar you see at restaurants for sweetening your coffee or tea? Each sugar packet contains 6 grams of sugar and 25 calories. The list below describes how many packets are in some popular foods. Look at the "nutritional facts" label if you are curious about other foods. Where the labels reads "sugars" divide that number by six. That will tell you how many packets of sugar are in that food item.

Soda pop (1 can) – 6.5 packets
Chocolate syrup (2 Tablespoons) – 6 packets
Gelatin (1/2 cup) – 5 packets

Pancake syrup (2 Tablespoons) – 7 packets
3 butterscotch candies – 2 packets
19 gummy or sour bears – 4 packets
Sugar wheat puff cereal (3/4 cup) – 2.5 packets
Cereal fruit bar – 3 packets
Muffin (large, store bought) – 3 packets

You can keep yourself away from these added sugars by choosing naturally sweet foods. Appreciate the wholesome goodness of fresh fruits and whole grains.

43.

YOU ARE A NUT!

How many times have you heard this phrase in your life? Though a "nutty" person may be strange or peculiar in nature, the food item known as a nut is of optimal yet somewhat peculiar nutrition. Nuts are wholesome healthy little bits of nutrition that you should recognize as necessary smart disease preventing food choices. However they are small little nuggets richly packed with calories. You must watch your consumption of them and not eat them by the handfuls.

Nuts are a remarkable snacking recommendation for athletes. If you are an athlete your body demands for high-energy food. Energy in food is measured in units called calories. Calories are what give our body energy. Nuts are *high* in calories. Thus they are perfect snacks for active people on the go. They are convenient, they do not spoil and most of all supply a delicious crunch.

Some nuts are rich in zinc. This is great for the immune system, appetite and skin. Cashews contain a high amount of zinc. Add vegetables, rice and sauce to make a popular Asian dish known as cashew chicken. Almonds provide a plentiful source of magnesium. Do you have high blood pressure? Magnesium is a mineral associated with regulating blood pressure. There is a significant amount of calcium in almonds and hazelnuts.

What about the fat in nuts? Yes, it is true; nuts are a high source of fat. But fat is not a nutrient we should totally eliminate from the diet. Fat is essential in the diet. Fat has positive attributes we rarely notice amidst all of the negative hype we hear. Do you want strong healthy shiny hair? How about healthy glowing skin? Fat is a nutrient contributing to many of the physical attributes we regard as attractive. However, too much fat in the diet can reverse the positive attributes fat brings to the body.

The fat is the healthy good fat we should eat for a healthy heart. A rich amount of the good fat, mono-unsaturated fat, is more desirable than a very low-fat diet. If you eat a diet rich in the good fat you will have a healthier blood cholesterol profile. You'll be better off than people who eat very low fat. Your HDL's (stands for high density lipoprotein) will be higher. Having high HDL's is most desirable. These "strong" lipoproteins are made of a small amount of lipid but a large amount of protein. Because the HDL's are so strong they have special duties in the body. One duty is to latch onto the bad fats and exit them out of your system.

How many nuts should you eat per day? Aim for eating two servings of these good fats a day. What is a serving? One ounce or two tablespoons of nuts a day will fulfill a nut serving. A good way to guesstimate an ounce is the same as the size of your thumb. The packet of nuts you receive on an airplane is one ounce in weight. It is about a quarter of a handful of nuts. Not a whole lot!

Being a nut is not so bad after all. You should not be offended to be considered a "nut" once in a while. Especially now that you are aware of all of the rich nutrients nuts supply our body with.

44.

ACHIEVING YOUR MONEY'S WORTH AT A BUFFET

How many of you have mixed feelings about buffets? Do you feel like you have to eat to get your money's worth? On average, buffet prices range from $6 to $40. There are ways to eat your money's worth *without* messing up your healthy eating plan. Be leery of temptation. Realize the pleasure of biting into delicious tasting food is nothing in comparison to feeling great about your body. Here is some advice to take with you to your next smorgasbord:

> **Omelet bar** – You can make a healthy omelet. Ask if egg substitutes are available or an omelet made of egg whites only. This will cut down on about 15 grams of fat. Skip the cheese in the omelet and replace it with vegetables like tomatoes, green pepper, spinach, tasty onions and celery pieces. Top the omelet off with salsa if available. Pepper the omelet and enjoy.

> **Soups** – Avoid the creamed soups. Creamed soups have many calories and fat grams. Instead go with the clear broth soups such as vegetable soup, chicken noodle, minestrone, and beef and vegetable barley. Tomato soup is also a good choice unless it is made with cream instead of water. If the soup looks dark red like catsup, it's probably safe for your healthy eating plan.

Hot Food – Take only three selections instead of having a bite of everything. Choose a lean meat entrée such as a chicken breast. Pull the skin off and flavor by squeezing a lemon wedge over top. Find a cooked vegetable you like. Flavor with a bit of olive oil from the salad bar and a grinding of fresh pepper. Choose a starch to compliment your two healthy choices. You can select a baked potato, brown rice, or a slice of whole wheat bread.

Fruit bar – This is a great place to get your dessert. Choose citrus fruits for Vitamin C. Try some berries or frozen fruit to top a healthy bowl of cereal at breakfast. Have one small glass of fruit juice.

Dessert – Make sure you take only one dessert. Frozen yogurt is a fabulous choice that includes Vitamin D and Calcium. Limit yourself to ½ cup.

Drinks – Have a glass of water with a lemon wedge. If you want something more special to drink, try a glass of seltzer water with a twist of lime. Have a cup of black coffee or tea if you wish. No calories there.

You are setting yourself up for temptation anytime you enter an all-you-can-eat buffet. Resist going up to the buffet for seconds. The second helping never tastes as good as the first anyhow. And most importantly, be on your guard!

45.

UNDERSTANDING DIABETES

Do you believe diabetes doesn't pertain to you or anyone you know? Maybe you think it is a disease you are exempt from. Perhaps medical information bores you. Whatever the case may be understand this; health experts estimate that approximately 6 million people have diabetes and do not know it!

There are two types of Diabetes - Type 1 Diabetes and Type 2 Diabetes. Type 1 Diabetes is an inborn disease. Type 2 Diabetes is a disease contracted later in life. It is usually caused by both genetics and being overweight.

People with diabetes cannot absorb sugar from food. There are two different reasons for this; hence Type 1 and Type 2. In a non-diabetic, the nutrients from food are digested and absorbed into the blood stream. The hormone insulin allows for these nutrients to be absorbed. This allows the non-diabetic to function throughout the day.

The Type 1 Diabetic does not release insulin. This is why Type 1 Diabetics take insulin injections. The insulin allows the Type 1 diabetic to absorb nutrients properly. Type 1 Diabetes accounts for five to ten percent of all diabetes cases. Most cases are diagnosed before the age of thirty. Symptoms include excessive thirst, frequent urination, and unexplainable weight loss. Type 2 Diabetes occurs most often in people over the age of thirty. Ninety percent to ninety-five percent of diabetes cases are Type 2. Eighty percent of these people are obese.

It is possible that the extra weight inhibits the body from functioning properly in Type 2. Insulin is not secreted as a normal person's is. The cell receptors that detect insulin do not respond anymore. This is why the Type

2 Diabetic is not treated with insulin injections as Type 1 is. The cell receptors aren't detecting the insulin anymore so there is no reason to inject the body with it.

A small reduction in body weight for the Type 2 Diabetic may decrease the extremity of this disease. Being diagnosed Type 2 Diabetic is extra motivation to lose weight. If you are Type 2 Diabetic you have to control your diabetes through your diet. Fortunately, the diet is a wonderful well-balanced plan that is appropriate for anyone. This diet can be used to control diabetes yet it also can be followed to prevent obesity. A Registered Dietitian can make the perfect diet for you depending on your height, age, weight, and activity level. The following is an example of a diabetic diet:

Breakfast:
1 whole grain frozen waffle
½ English muffin
½ cup prunes
1 cup skim milk

Morning snack:
1 slice of sourdough bread

Lunch:
1 Roast Beef Sandwich with lettuce, tomato
1 tsp. mayonnaise
Diet Coke
½ c. chocolate ice cream

Afternoon Snack:
Chicken broth

Dinner:

3 oz. slice of meatloaf
½ c. instant mashed potatoes made with milk (no fat added)
½ c. three bean salad
1 slice of rye bread
½ c. steamed asparagus
½. cup fresh chopped pineapple

Evening snack:
1 c. canned tangerines

Notice how it is evenly balanced throughout the day. Fifty to sixty percent of the calories come from carbohydrate, twenty to twenty-five percent from protein and fewer than thirty percent from fat. Additionally, fewer than ten percent of the fat calories are from saturated fat. This meal plan is a good idea for *anyone*, not just a diabetic.

46.

THINK OF "WORKING OUT" LIKE "GOING OUT"

Do you cringe at the thought of working out? Does it sound better to spend your free time out on the town? Imagine that you have plans to spend the evening with your favorite person. You have been looking forward to this all week. Envision how this makes you feel.

This is how it made me feel. I envisioned laughing, smiling, talking, meeting new people, casually drinking refreshing liquids, bright colors, dancing, music, and excitement. I definitely had something to look forward to.

These are the same words that describe how you can feel when you work out. You let loose when you work out. If you bring a friend there is laughter, smiles and conversation. You usually will meet new people. You can enjoy refreshing ice-cold water. The atmosphere is bright. There is always energizing music. Once you begin to move, your endorphin (feel-good) hormones are released. You feel awesome!

Working out and going out are very similar activities. Why should you view working out as a burden? There are ways to be entertained while working out. Choose an activity you enjoy. Do not run if you don't like to. Choose another activity like biking or power walking. If you hate weightlifting, take up tai chi or yoga – both are awesome activities that improve muscle tone, posture, balance and flexibility.

Exercise is more than just a way to burn calories; it's a way to have fun. Choose an activity that you like to do. Do your activity when you feel like going out. The more you go out the better.

47.

TAKE OUT THE GARBAGE

Losing weight is not only a physical battle, but psychological also. One must set aside time to work on the mental self. Perhaps incorporate this time into your workout. You can use yoga as not only physical but also mental and spiritual exercise. Yoga is recommended for weight loss and is a stress reliever.

Try to meditate while jogging or walking. Your route can be mapped into four sections. Concentrate on a different thought during each section of the jog. This is a way to make the time go by quicker! You will also be more efficient because you are multi-tasking. Many people can't relax themselves enough to sit and meditate for half an hour. Incorporating it into your exercise routine is better than not at all.

Yoga is designed to release the physical and mental stresses we endure each day. It is a way to take out the garbage. You will feel your body relax in areas you did not realize were tense. You may be reluctant to deal with these tensions. However it is vital to reaching your goals. Here are a couple of ways to release negative thoughts and replace them with positive:

> **The Thankful Meditation** – Begin by taking deep breaths in and out. Breathe deeply and fill all of the space in your abdominal cavity. Begin thinking about how good your life is. Even if you have a difficult time finding the good in your life, you can always find something. After about 5 minutes of your good realization, switch your thoughts carefully to what is troubling you. Think of the situation. Do not blame anyone including you. Just think

of troubling times. Once you've found stress, positively begin to think of ways to deal with this it. Have an open mind. Try to envision yourself as a mediator. Look from the outside into the situation. Seeing the stress from the outside will give you an entirely new perspective. This is a time to grow inwardly and see how you can approach the situation differently. After ten minutes of meditation, thank yourself for allowing the time to deal with pressure.

The Mantra Meditation – Mantra is the practice of repeating a word over and over again with each breath you take. Begin with a journal. Write down many positive adjectives that describe you. Be aware of how you are feeling when you do this. Some of the words will be how you feel about yourself. Others may be good words that people have said about you that you did not realize. Pick the word that makes you feel best. Repeat this word several times as you breathe deeply in and out. Meditate on you and that word for at least 5 minutes. Now switch your focus to the first letter of this word. Think of positive sentences about yourself that all begin with the first letter. Choose the one sentence that perks you up. Now repeat in a mantra as you breathe deeply in and out.

Be disciplined and continue this practice daily. You may choose one meditation to concentrate on, or do both by alternating days. You may even choose a different meditation that is more suitable for you. It is important to do this regularly to be effective. As you reach for your nutritional and fitness goals, use meditations to guide you and lift you up.

Relax! Don't let yourself feel rushed. This takes practice. Building your meditation endurance is similar to building your aerobic endurance. You may only be able to take ten minutes out of your day to start with. After a year, you could be spending an hour. You may encounter a momentous time in your meditations. Do not quit. Liven your meditations with different practices other than the ones you were doing. You can find ideas from other books and the Internet. I wish you the best...and don't forget to take out the garbage!

48.

MEAL REPLACEMENTS

If you had the choice between the following two dinners, which diet plan would you choose?

Diet Plan A – Whole Foods
Tossed greens with ½ Tablespoon low fat dressing
3 oz. Grilled lemon chicken breast
1 c. Strawberries with a small amount whipped topping
1 Multivitamin

Diet Plan B – Packaged Foods
1 Diet Shake

Both of the dinners supply the body with the same amount of calories along with an adequate supply of vitamins and minerals. Aside from the obvious difference that one provides substantial food and the other one is a cool beverage, there are other variances.

Dinner B is just as tasty as drinking a nice cold refreshing glass of chocolate milk. The size of your portion is controlled with Diet Plan B. It is convenient because there is no thinking involved. However, this diet plan is challenging to stay committed to because all of the meals are the same.

Dinner A is a more appealing option for those of you who prefer to *eat* your calories as opposed to drinking them. This is important for meal satisfaction! However, with Diet Plan A you may have to resist the urge to take a larger portion than what is allocated.

You are eating real food with Dinner A. You might be able to lose weight by drinking shakes everyday but how will you function in the real world? When will you learn what menu choices at the restaurants are laden with fat? How do you develop the resistance to devour that whole basket of chips? Diet Plan A teaches you the skills to make healthy choices for a lifetime.

Another example of meal replacements is energy bars. The original target audience of these bars was for athletes involved in activity for longer than one and a half hours at a time. It is the food equivalent to a sports drink. The bar supplies quick energy so athletes can finish their performance. People misuse the bars for a splurge of "energy". What these people need to realize is the energy received from these bars is no different than the energy received from an apple, a stalk of celery, or a container of yogurt. Energy is calories and calories are energy. The same amount of calories is in both, but one is easier to pack on the go.

Wholesome food in moderation is by far the best choice for weight control. It is healthier to eat normal food in moderation combined with exercise as opposed to yo-yo dieting with monotonous meal replacements.

49.

LOSING FAT...NOT MUSCLE

Losing fat and not muscle is a common concern among athletic individuals. This should be a concern for anyone who is losing weight. Muscle is our calorie burning mechanism. The more muscle you have the more calories you burn. You should maximize fat loss and minimize muscle loss when losing weight. Be aware that you will typically lose some muscle. Here are some things to consider:

Lose Less Weight Per Week - A slower, more drawn out process will help maintain more muscle storage in your body. Losing 1 to 2 pounds per week is optimal for maintaining more muscle. Many dieters aren't concerned about conserving maximum muscle mass. These dieters want to lose weight faster.

Less Intense Activities - You can use moderately intense aerobic activity combined with anaerobic strength training. Moderately intense activities include walking, biking, gymnastics, golf, dancing and hiking. Perform your favorite moderate activity four days per week. Eventually try increasing to one hour per session. Moderately intense activity helps to burn a higher percentage of body fat. Intense exercise causes you to burn less fat. The anaerobic exercise should be some form of weight training or toning exercises. You can do weight training two to three times per week.

Dietary Protein - Protein is overrated in terms of intake. It is *not* true that more protein intake causes more muscle development. Exercising your muscles is what promotes muscle development. The average person needs 0.4 grams of protein per pound of body weight per day. The active person needs 1 gram of protein per pound of body weight per day. This is not difficult to obtain through normal eating.

For example:

A 125-pound active female who exercises 15 hours per week has higher protein needs as a result of her high activity level.

125 pounds X 1 gram protein = 125 grams of protein recommended

125 grams protein X 4 calories/gram protein = 500 calories

This female needs about 2000 calories to support her active body. (2000 calories may be too high for some inactive females. Use 2500 calories as a general number for males.)

What percent of her diet is protein at 500 calories of protein per day? 500/2000=25%

This female eats a healthy diet consisting of: 50% carbohydrate, 25% fat and 25% protein.

Try to calculate this for yourself considering your weight and activity level. Record everything you eat for a day. Add up the protein grams and see how much protein you really are eating. You can look-up the protein content on the food labels. Remember that one ounce of animal meat has 7 grams of protein. Are you close to your recommended amount? You can make adjustments in your diet to get better results.

50.

NUTRITION - A FOUNTAIN OF YOUTH

Someone once asked me if there was a way to eat to prevent aging. If there was, I'm sure it would be no secret and we would all know about it. There are small actions you can take to keep the aging process to a minimum. These little health tricks can keep you looking, feeling, and being young.

First thing you need to do is kick the nicotine habit. This habit adds years to your face making your skin wrinkle faster. Your skin tone and coloring is much healthier once you stop this habit. Smoking damages the cardiovascular system and lung capacity.

Exercise is a major contributor to youthfulness. It is not true that you are going to lose your stamina and muscle tone once over the age of thirty. Some people use age as an excuse to stop exercising. A major reason why I calculate calorie needs lower for a person as he/she ages is because the average person becomes less active. There are three dimensions to exercise, which keep your body in top condition:

> **Aerobics** –It is best that aerobic exercise be done for 40 minutes at least three times per week.

> **Flexibility** – Though many people skip this part of the workout it is just as important as any other workout segment. Stretch your hamstrings, calves, gluteus maximums, back, abdominal, and arms. Stretching is essential in making your muscles more limber. People who incorporate stretching into their regular workout routine

are less prone to accidents. Stretching also will improve your balance.

Strength – People lose their strength because they decrease their activity level. It is possible to keep your muscles toned through age 60.

Consume whole grains and fruits and vegetables. It is probable that nutrients can improve skin's appearance. Eat a diet rich in vitamins and minerals for a healthy glow.

Lastly, think positively! When you think positively it is less stressful on the body. Did you know it actually takes more muscles to frown then it does to smile? Save your muscle work and energy for exercising and turn that frown into a smile.

51.

CREATIVE AND CONVENIENT

Frozen food is tremendously beneficial to our hurried lifestyles. However, the food inside the frozen package may be short of delivering a completely balanced meal to your body. Some of the frozen foods have high amounts of fat while others include no vegetables.

When choosing frozen entrees, check the nutrition label. An average person needs about twenty to thirty percent of his/her calories to be from fat. That is about 60-80 grams of fat per day. Most lean entrées deliver lower amounts of fat than their counterparts.

Complete your meal by adding whole foods to your frozen entrée. Include a cool glass of skim milk, one half cup of green veggies, maybe a slice of whole grain bread (optional) and fruit for dessert. This is an example of a well-balanced frozen entrée meal.

Other ideas of fast and easy foods to prepare include canned soups, oatmeal, and sandwiches. Vegetable, bean and lentil soups are terrific ideas for a boost in vitamins and minerals. For breakfast, oatmeal provides a quick inexpensive meal, filled with fiber. Add milk and fruit and you're good to go. For lunch, a peanut butter sandwich is convenient and tasty. Instead of jam, sprinkle some dried fruit and chopped celery within the sandwich. It will give the sandwich extra crunch.

Being busy is not an excuse for eating unhealthy. Take advantage of convenience foods. Be creative and add your own touches to make it a completely balanced meal!

52.

NUTRITION AND INSURANCE

Nutrition is the cornerstone to good health. Good nutrition actually is influential in preventing six of the top ten most common causes of death in America today. If people started caring more about their nutrition early in life, they could bypass future problems. Wouldn't you rather avoid being in the hospital for three days due to a cardiac arrest? You can save time, money, heartache and complications by thinking ahead and living healthy.

Unfortunately, it's not that easy. There is an abundance of nutritional information available to us from the media, Internet, authors, friends and health professionals. Who do we believe? To learn the facts of nutrition the professionals that people need to seek out are *registered dietitians*. These are the "nutrition experts" recognized by the medical community.

Insurance firms would be wise to cover nutritional counseling. The insurance companies could save several thousand dollars in medical costs. Unfortunately, insurance does *not* cover most nutritional counseling. There are rare cases in which insurance does cover nutritional counseling. Most often it is *after* the medical problem has already occurred. From an economical and health standpoint, this does not make sense.

Why isn't nutrition counseling covered by insurance? This is a very touchy subject for us registered dietitians. We care about *you* and your health. We want very badly for insurance companies to change their ways. The American Dietetic Association is trying with great effort to change things for you.

Nutrition counseling is covered if you are diabetic or have kidney disease. It helps to have a doctor's referral, a letter backing this referral up from the M.D. along with a receipt and letter from the dietitian describing her nutritional assessment.

53.

NUTRITION FOR WOMEN OF CHILDBEARING-AGE

Becoming pregnant is a phase in life not to be taken lightly, especially in regards to nutrition. The pregnant woman will be supporting the life of not only herself, but also the life growing inside her. Therefore, foods must be highly nutritious and calorie needs must be met. A woman contemplating pregnancy should ask herself these questions:

- Do I eat nutritiously for health as opposed to maintaining my figure?

- Will I take the time to eat and deliver nutrients to my body and my baby as needed?

- Am I willing to choose foods that are high in important nutrients as opposed to eating foods that only taste good?

After a woman has thought about this among other aspects then the decision to become pregnant can be made. Some women do not consider the ramifications of becoming pregnant. They are more concerned with their body image. She must feed the baby and herself proper nutrients. Just as important, she must be ready to teach her child healthy eating habits along with displaying a positive body image. The child will emulate these desirable behaviors.

In a recent study done with pregnant women of all ages, there were significant deficiencies in several nutrients. Here are some suggestions of foods offering a rich supply of each particular nutrient:

Calcium – Includes yogurt, Swiss cheese, cheddar cheese and fat-free milk.

Magnesium – Spinach, peanut butter, black-eyed peas, tofu, sunflower seeds, halibut, cashews and artichokes have magnesium.

Zinc – Oysters, lean sirloin steak, lean ground beef, crab, and turkey (dark meat) each include zinc.

Iron – You will find iron in lean sirloin, lean ground beef, skinless chicken breast, lean pork, fortified breakfast cereals, pumpkin seeds, canned clams, tofu, soybean nuts, beef liver, parsley, and shrimp.

Folate – Oranges, orange juice, spinach, black-eyed peas, lentils, pinto beans, garbanzo beans, peanuts, and okra each contain folate. Also, enriched grain products must be fortified with folic acid.

Vitamin D – Includes egg yolks, liver, fatty fish, margarine and fortified milk.

Vitamin E – Almonds, wheat germ, peanut butter, soybean oil, corn oil, sunflower seeds, and tofu have vitamin E.

It is vital for a woman to get plenty of folate early in the pregnancy. Folate is the vitamin responsible for making important contributions to rapidly growing cells. That is what is occurring in pregnancy. Neural tube birth defects such as spina bifida are more likely to arise if the expecting mother does not ingest adequate folate in the first trimester. Women taking a folate supplement one month prior to becoming pregnant and throughout the first trimester are much less prone to these birth defects. It is recommended that *all* women of childbearing age consume adequate amounts of folate because many women are not aware when they are pregnant. Talk to your doctor about your folate needs before and during your pregnancy.

The moderately active pregnant woman requires an extra 300 calories per day. Consuming an extra 300 calories can be quite easy. Simply add one food from each food group (fruit, starch, vegetable, milk and one ounce of lean meat). You may be surprised to know that the lactating mother actually needs more calories than the expecting mother.

Weight gain during pregnancy is inevitable. The amount varies depending on the weight before pregnancy. For a woman who is at a healthy weight, gaining 25 to 35 pounds is sufficient. An underweight woman should gain between 28 and 40 pounds. The overweight woman should gain no more than 15 to 25 pounds. Under no circumstances should a pregnant woman try to lose weight during any term of her pregnancy.

Does the average 25 to 35 pound weight gain seem like a lot to you? If a typical baby weighs 7.5 pounds, where is all the extra weight coming from? The extra weight comes from changes that occur in the body to support the growing fetus. There is extra blood, development of the placenta, uterus, and breasts. Some fat is stored in the expecting mother for energy needs during the actual birthing process.

Many women wonder if exercising during pregnancy is allowed. Check with your physician to get approval first. Exercise is recommended for those in a healthy pregnancy. Consider the advantages to staying active during the term:

- Easier labor
- Outlet for stress
- Ability to lose weight after the pregnancy
- Decreases chance of gestational diabetes

A pregnant woman can improve her fitness level in the nine months of her term. She should listen closely to her body and know when to stop. Activities that are recommended are ones with less contact, fewer jarring motions and ones that maintain the body at a relatively cool temperature. Good exercises include walking, stationary bike riding, swimming and water aerobics. Do not do exercises such as riding a bike outdoors, step aerobics and volleyball.

This nutritional information will help guide you to deliver a healthy baby. You can find a dietitian near you at http://www.eatright.org to recommend an optimal diet for your personal needs.

54.

THE BUZZ ON CAFFEINE

Do you choose caffeine beverages instead of calcium-rich beverages? Not having dairy products can be unhealthy. In addition, having three cups of coffee per day decreases absorption of calcium. If you consume caffeine be strict about having three to four servings of dairy per day.

Caffeine helps relieve pain from headaches by restricting the blood flow in the brain. Most aspirin contain caffeine. However, just as caffeine consumption relieves pain from headaches it can also cause headaches when you stop. The increase of blood in the head is what causes the throbbing sensation.

Caffeine does not hinder iron absorption. Coffee and tea contain polyphenols, which inhibit the absorption of plant-based iron.

Caffeine may enhance long-term memory. Researchers found that consuming caffeine after learning may help enhance long-term memory.

Caffeine enhances performance in some athletes. You may conclude that possibly there are advantages to caffeine since the Olympic Committee disqualifies athletes with large doses of caffeine.

Caffeine will increase blood sugars. Caffeine may not be the healthiest option of all foods when low in blood sugar. However it is an option when there is nothing else around. Caffeine raises the metabolism. Some weight-loss pills have caffeine to increase calorie burning.

Do you have problems with anxiety? Caffeine will magnify the problem. Caffeine's effect on the nervous system mimics and increases the feelings of anxiety. Are you hypertensive? Caffeine increases the heart rate slightly, which is an effect you need not engage in.

You make your own choices. That is the bottom line. Caffeine has a different degree of effect on each of us.

55.

I LOVE FOOD TOO MUCH TO EAT HEALTHY

I don't know a single person who doesn't love food! Someone once asked me, "If you love food, how can you give up eating delicious foods such as French fries?" I haven't and neither should you! I just eat them on occasion when my body is truly craving it.

Are you envious of people that can turn down a rich piece of chocolate cake? Do you wish you had the same control? I use to experience this. I didn't feel too good about myself after the pounds began to add up. I became overweight. Although I loved food, I loved myself too. I decided to make a change. I started to follow a program similarly structured to the Food Guide Pyramid. I made adjustments to my eating habits without feeling deprived. I was still able to enjoy food. Instead of eating brownies, cake or ice cream every night for dessert, I would alternate between oranges, apples, sugar-free pudding and once in a while a slice of cake. At fast food joints I began opting for the grilled chicken salads instead of the hamburger and fries. I was beginning to establish an appreciation for foods on the bottom side of the Pyramid as opposed to appreciating only the top half of the Pyramid.

You too can establish this sense of enjoyment. You *can* train yourself to appreciate healthy foods. You will be favoring your whole self as opposed to only your taste buds and appetite.

If you do love rich succulent foods and you would like to devour them more frequently, exercise! Let's say you walk everyday for half an hour. Your roommate sits and watches TV during your walk. Your roommate and you eat a half-cup of ice cream every night. That half hour walk is enough exercise to burn the calories from the ice cream you ate. Your friend will gain a pound a month, while you will maintain.

Be aware that everyone loves food just as you do. Our bodies are made to feel satisfied after consuming delicious rich foods. A healthy person has established a discipline of knowing when and how much to indulge. Indulging only occasionally makes the scrumptious food taste all the more better. Only this time the love for the food is controllable.

56.

I'M TOO BUSY!

Are you too busy to exercise and watch what you eat? I hear this a lot. It seems everyone is too busy. There a few people who do manage to fit health into their lifestyle. What is the difference between the busy people who make time to exercise and eat right and those who do not? Its priorities. For some, fitness and health is on their priorities list. For others it is not. Both parties are equally as busy; they just have different priorities. You've seen news clips of Bill Clinton, former President of the United States, taking a jog haven't you?

Eating healthy takes very little extra time. You will spend some time educating yourself. By now, you have read enough chapters from this book to get you by. Healthy food is available everywhere you go. You are probably already quicker at knowing how to choose healthy food. You can still eat fast food. Every fast food restaurant offers a variety of healthy selections. When in doubt, have one of the salad choices (except the taco salad). You can pour a little low calorie dressing on top and order a skim milk. You can order a side salad with a grilled chicken breast sandwich. Request the sauce on the side. That way you can control the amount that you consume. You can have fat-free muffins and cereal if you like to have a fast breakfast.

The fact of the matter is that you make time to do what is important to you. I try never to tell anyone that I was "too busy". If our former president had the time to exercise and eat healthy, than we all do!

57.

VEGETARIAN FOR THE DAY

Have you ever wanted to try vegetarianism? Do you think you would feel satisfied without eating meat? Being a vegetarian does not always mean refraining from eating animal meat. There are different types of vegetarians.

Semi vegetarians - Also known as partial vegetarians. These people exclude only some animal derived foods from their diet. Most people in this category eliminate red meat and consume poultry and seafood.

Lacto-ovo-vegetarians - People who exclude animal, seafood, and bird flesh from their diet.

Lacto vegetarians - People who include milk products but exclude animal flesh and eggs from their diet.

Vegans - These people exclude all products derived from animals. For example, a vegan would refrain from eating a cake if it was made with eggs and butter.

All four styles of vegetarianism can be healthy. Excluding foods from a diet makes it more challenging to eat well-balanced meals. If you exclude dairy, you need to make a special effort to acquire Vitamin D, Vitamin B12, and calcium from other sources. One cup of leafy greens added to a diet provides calcium, Vitamins D, iron and zinc. You can supplement with a multi-vitamin to ensure you are receiving B12 and other nutrients.

Many people wonder if vegetarians receive enough protein. People do not realize that most foods contain protein. Vegetarians are able to consume protein in sufficient amounts by doing their nutrition research.

There are several vegetarians who eat a rather unhealthy diet. Cutting out animal products from a diet does not justify eating more junk food. Ordering a mound of French fries with a side salad, then eating two cupcakes afterwards is an example of unhealthy vegetarianism. Whether vegetarian or not, you must still make an effort to eat healthy with plenty of produce and whole grains.

There are advantages of vegetarianism. Vegetarians tend to experience lower blood pressure and less chance of suffering from heart disease and cancer. It is a great idea for you to be vegetarian one day a week. Consider these tasty possibilities:

- Whole grain pasta with tomato sauce and Parmesan cheese sprinkled on top.

- Bean burrito wrapped in a whole-wheat tortilla filled with low-fat cheese, lettuce, low-fat sour cream, tomatoes and onions.

- Pita with Feta cheese, olives, lettuce, tomatoes and cucumbers drizzled with olive oil.

- Veggie burger on whole-wheat bun with oven baked fries

- Baked potato filled with bean chili and low-fat cheddar.

58.

HOLIDAY STRATEGIES

They say it's the most wonderful time of the year. What would November and December be without the holidays? The food is fantastic! That could be why the average American gains weight during this time. To advert from this weight gain, focus on other aspects of the holidays. If you can do that, your chances of gaining weight will diminish.

Weight gain is gradual so use these tips all season long. The tips are divided into three different categories: food, fitness, and psychological.

Food:

- Don't eat a huge breakfast on Thanksgiving. Budget your eating. Consume a light breakfast like a glass of 1% milk or a piece of toast with peanut butter. If you become hungry later on at night, pop some popcorn for a light snack.

- Substitute low-fat or non-fat products in recipes. Ex. Low-fat sour cream for dips, evaporated skimmed milk for heavy cream in sauces, low-fat cheese in casseroles and cheese trays.

- Stay away from high-fat sauces. Rely on salsa, nonfat yogurt, flavored vinegar, vegetable purees, fresh lemon juice, or crushed tomatoes to bring flavor to your food.

- When it's time for guests to leave, bring out the plastic bags and *give food away*! Don't keep all of it in the refrigerator to tempt you for the next couple of days.

- Give leftover desserts to your spouse to take to work.

- Clean the kitchen without nibbling.

- Eat slowly and savor every bite. Talking during mealtime will help you eat more slowly. Drink water between mouthfuls to clear your palette and enjoy each piece more.

- Do you really need 2 rolls, a half-cup of mashed potatoes, stuffing, sweet potatoes, *and* corn? That's a lot of starch! Limit your intake to what you *really* want. For example, a reasonable choice would be ½ cup of stuffing and one roll. If you can't give up everything, take one to two tablespoons worth of each starchy dish. Grab a roll, some turkey and go sit down. Enjoy!

- Stop eating when you are full even if this means leaving food on your plate. Others will be less likely to force more food on you.

- When watching football try to keep your hands full of items other than food. Instead of having a handful of potato chips, replace it with confetti to throw on the touchdowns!

- Keep yourself busy. Don't just linger at the table stuffing unwanted calories into your mouth. Go play a game with the kids, go outside and play basketball, or read a book to your favorite cousin. Take your mind off food.

Exercise:

- Exercise everyday during the holidays. This will keep your metabolism running at high levels!

- Try an interval training class at your local gym. You will burn more calories from doing intervals plus feel so proud of yourself.

- If you normally have a maid clean your house, burn some extra calories and do it yourself.

Psychological:

- Take a moment and picture how you want the day to go for you nutritionally. Decide how you are going to keep from becoming uncomfortably full.

- Realize that Thanksgiving Day is not the last day to eat. If you are too full to eat dessert, there's always tomorrow. Save it for when you can enjoy it more.

- Vent your feelings days before in a journal to prevent yourself from becoming aggravated at family gatherings.

- Remind yourself that you are eating this way because you are learning new nutritional habits, which you will keep for a lifetime. You are not doing this to torture yourself. Don't lose focus of the light at the end of the tunnel during the holidays. Remember the reason why you are changing your eating habits, whether it is to lose weight or lower your cholesterol.

- Rehearse saying, "no thank you" so you can politely decline food offers.

- When taking bites, ask yourself, "Do I really want this?" Make sure you are eating because you are hungry, not just to eat.

You can still strive for your nutrition goals during the holidays. Instead of viewing the holidays as a time to allow your diet to slip, make it a time to teach yourself discipline!

59.

THINK POSITIVELY!

Think positively about nutrition. Think about what you *should* eat rather than what you shouldn't. There are several healthy foods. Some of them have a higher concentrate of nutrients. Here are ten food items that you should consume several times per week:

Legumes – Beans! Beans are full of fiber, low in fat, and high in minerals, vitamins, carbohydrates and protein.

Tip: The next time you eat Mexican, order a bean burrito.

Onions – Onions contain disease-fighting chemicals called antioxidants. Onions are 90 percent water and thus they are very low in calories.

Tip: Putting onions in a salad will add a lot of flavor. You will not need to use much salad dressing.

Skim milk – If drinking skim milk makes you cringe, ½% or 1% is fine. Milk has riboflavin (vitamin B2), Vitamin D and calcium. Calcium is essential for bone mineralization. It helps prevent osteoporosis.

Tip: Sugar-free pudding mixed with skim milk is a delicious healthy dessert. Top it with whipped topping for extra low fat flavor.

Oranges – Oranges have disease-fighting chemicals in them called antioxidants. They are rich in vitamin C. These chemicals can prevent you from getting cancer or the common cold. Oranges can also be consumed to shorten the duration of your cold.

Tip: A magnificent morning treat! Slice a small whole-wheat bagel in half and spread on one tablespoon of low-fat cream cheese. Top the bagel off by placing orange segments on the cream cheese.

Salmon – Cold-water fish are rich in omega-3 fatty acids. Omega-3 fatty acids keep your cholesterol at healthy levels. Salmon is also a lean source of protein.

Tip: Don't always order a steak. Most steak house menus contain a salmon dinner. Order salmon instead of the prime rib.

Tomato juice – Tomatoes are a fruit thus you should think of tomato juice as a fruit juice, rather than the less appetizing vegetable juice. It is lower in calories than most fruit juices.

Tip: Try red beer. It's a German tradition. It's made from one-third spicy tomato-juice (or Bloody Mary mix) and two-thirds light beer. It is very in low calories – 95 calories per 12 oz.

Oatmeal – Oatmeal is high in fiber. It lowers cholesterol and makes your stomach full longer.

Tip: Add spice with nutmeg and/or cinnamon, dried fruit and/or fresh fruit, nuts, and a teaspoon of vanilla extract for flavor.

Lemons/limes – This is another antioxidant fruit. Lemons and limes are acidic. Eating acids help fight germs.

Tip: Add a squeeze of lemon or lime instead of using salt for flavor.

Garlic – Garlic is also a disease-fighter, which lowers the risk of getting cancer and heart disease.

Tip: Bake a garlic head. Spread the soft cloves on to slices of whole wheat bread.

Sweet potatoes/yams – Orange vegetables contain vitamin A and beta-carotene. Vitamin A is important in eyesight, skin condition and disease prevention. Beta-carotene is a powerful antioxidant.

Tip: Top your sweet potato with light margarine and cinnamon.

Eating is an opportunity to fill your body with as many nutrients as possible. Eat these foods often and you will reach that goal.

60.

TRY NEW THINGS

Are you afraid to try something new when it comes to eating? This can be scary, especially if you are picky.

You could be missing out on nutrients unique to foods you don't eat. You might not like mushy foods, such as oatmeal. Instead you eat toast every morning. I'm not knocking toast. It has its own distinctive goodness. Have oatmeal in lieu of toast just once a week. This will increase your nutrient consumption. A bowl of oatmeal has 4 grams of fiber. You need 20 grams of fiber per day. Fiber reduces cholesterol levels. Oatmeal will make you fuller than toast. Not convinced? Be creative! Add zest with dried cranberries or even chocolate chips. Use a flavor that is suitable for you.

As you grow older, your likes and dislikes change. When I was a child I did not like asparagus. Now I eat asparagus with no regard. Try a food you dislike. Your opinion may be different now. Here are some meal choices to broaden your horizons:

Bagel with Roasted Red Pepper and Hummus
Mango Chicken Salad
Gyro with Feta Cheese
Portabella Sandwich
Veggie Burger
Tomato Cilantro Couscous Salad
Macadamia Crusted Opah
Cobb Salad with Avocado

61.

MORE BANG FOR YOUR BUCK

Do you experience cognitive dissonance when you are selecting bread at the grocery store? The white bread is less expensive and it tastes better to you. The 100 percent whole wheat bread is healthy but it's double the price.

You may be saving money initially by buying the cheaper product. However you will not save in the long run. You want to be at your best possible health when you become older. You will avoid numerous trips to the doctor not to mention high health insurance costs and medications. These costs are much greater than the amount you save by eating less expensive food.

You want to get the most bang for your buck. Vegetables, fruits, whole grains, fish and low-fat dairy products are some great examples. These foods have lots of vitamins, minerals, fiber and phytochemicals. Here are some other shopping tips that will yield less hospital visits, fewer medical bills and less time in a hospital bed:

Read Nutrient Labels - Read the ingredient list. Is there a lot of sugar in the product? Notice the order of the ingredients. If sugar appears as one of the first few items, there is a large amount of sugar. Sugar is empty of any vitamins and minerals.

Compare Price – Don't just evaluate total cost. Compare price per ounce, per item, per gram, etc. This information is readily available and labeled at most grocers next to the total price label on the shelf.

Leave the chips - Don't buy foods that are going to damage your healthy nutrition plan. These foods can be a waste of money and waste of calories. For example, if you can't keep your hand out of the chip bag, just forget them.

Convenience Foods – Is buying pre-packaged food a cheaper option for you? It might be worth your time to make foods from scratch. Or it may not, especially if you have the money and you are short on free time. You can add fruits and vegetables to frozen dinners to make it more complete. Cooking can take some effort, but it is constructive fun effort.

Be wise and budget when you go grocery shopping. Choose money-savers, clip coupons and watch for sales. Just remember that your life and your health are most important.

62.

THE TABOO TIP TO WEIGHT CONTROL

Sex and weight maintenance – the two go hand and hand. Consider this. A female, let's name her Debbie, is 23 and *not* sexually active. Although she dates quite a bit, she refrains for moral and health reasons. Debbie absolutely *loves* rich chocolate desserts. The more caramel, fudge, and nuts the dessert has, the better. Debbie indulges in such a dessert once a day. Because Debbie is physically active most days of the week, she is not obese but would be considered slightly overweight.

Debbie's sister, recently married at age of 28, and is sexually active. She used to have the same cravings. Since then her cravings changed. The intense rich dessert craving decreased dramatically after a couple of weeks of sexual activity. Sex satisfies food cravings in some people. This made Debbie very curious.

Do not become sexually active just to eliminate your food cravings. With the scare of sexually transmitted diseases, that would be unhealthier than being obese! However, if you are married and have uncontrollable urges to eat food, analyze your sex life. How often do you participate in sexual activity with your spouse? Once a month is not enough! Try boosting that up to four to five times a week instead. Get creative. Revitalize your love!

Realize that food is just one part of life. Don't make it the center. We tend to be lazy at night. It's the same old routine - a bowl of ice cream and 3 hours of television and Internet. That is why we are over weight. There is more to life than food! Your relationship with your spouse is *extremely* important. Make love at least once for every three times you eat. You'll really be losing weight!

63.

SUPPLEMENT NOT SUBSTITUE

Should we take supplements? That is a question I'm frequently asked. Some dietitians believe all nutrients should be obtained through food. I believe it is a good idea to take a daily multi-vitamin to achieve the 100 percent Daily Value of all vitamins and minerals.

I also agree that you should receive most of your nutrition through food. When you receive your nutrients through food your body's absorption rate is higher than if it were through a supplement. Foods contain other disease fighting compounds that supplements do not. Vegetables and fruits not only carry vitamins and minerals they also contain some phytochemicals, which are only found in food. Phytochemicals keep us healthy by decreasing the risk of cardiovascular disease and cancer. Eat a diet based on vegetables, fruits and whole grains. Complete your meal with a lean protein source and low-fat dairy products. Doing so will supply your body with the needed vitamins and minerals. Your diet will be lower in fat and calories. Supplements should not take the place of healthy foods.

Beware to those of you shopping for a supplement. There are many supplements out there that make magical claims. There are also supplements that are expensive. These devious companies make a quick buck by fooling you into buying supplements that you do not need. Other supplements provide you with 1600 percent of your daily needs of Vitamin C! Your body will only use 100 percent of what it needs. Taking mega-doses of certain vitamins can be dangerous to your health.

64.

WHOLE GRAINS

Whole grains are a natural healthy choice. Choosing whole grains is difficult because it is rarely offered. You may not like the taste or the extra cost compared to white bread. You can elevate your wellness by eating whole grains.

I am sure you have heard of fiber, but really, what is fiber? Could you answer that question if someone asked you? Fiber is the part of plant foods that cannot be digested by the human body.

Whole grains are hearty. You will eat less and feel better. You could eat two servings of whole grain pasta and feel just as full as you would if you ate five servings of white pasta. Reducing your carbohydrate consumption is an added benefit.

Whole grain products contain a slightly larger amount of fat. Don't let this deter you from choosing whole grains. The amount of fat is insignificant and it's the healthy fat anyhow.

The grain of wheat is composed of three parts: the bran, endosperm and germ. The bran is the outer covering of the grain. This is where the fiber is. The bran also contains Vitamin B. The endosperm is the large middle part of the grain. It contains protein and carbohydrate. The germ is the smallest part of the grain. It is found in the center. It contains unsaturated fat; protein, iron and Vitamin B. White bread is made from the endosperm. Nutrients are eliminated in white bread. The FDA requires the food manufacturers to enrich white flour with nutrients lost during processing. However, fiber and phytochemicals are left out.

65.

A WEIGHT-LOSS SPONSOR

Have you ever thought about helping a family member or friend lose weight? You may not realize how much it forces you to become healthier. Your friend or family may want to lean on someone for nutritional help. However you will have to be a good role model in order to give them what they want.

You can show this person that it is possible to eat a delicious piece of chocolate cake and still have a slender fit body. It will be motivating for you to know that he/she will look up to you for healthy lifestyle changes.

Pick a friend, a brother or sister, a father or mother or even a cousin. Choose someone who has complained about his/her weight. Gently approach that person with an idea. Tell him/her that you are also unsatisfied with your own body and are working diligently on changing it. You can also say that you are just tickled about your new healthy eating habits. Tell this person that teaching him/her what you've learned would motivate you to stay on track. You will be able to help each other reach your goals.

Consider this if you don't want to feel pushy. What do you do when you see a fantastic movie? You tell people about it! The same goes for a new healthy eating plan. Do not be greedy and hide good health from those you love. Share, help, and teach them how you are learning to eat healthy!

You'll gain a perspective of being on the other side of the table when someone is lagging from his/her eating plan. You will both be able to keep each other accountable. This is perhaps the most import part of having a weight-loss sponsor.

66.

AN EXCUSE TO EAT CHOCOLATE?

Do you like chocolate? How often do you eat it? Here is the scoop on chocolate. Chocolate contains cancer-fighting antioxidants called polyphenols. In fact chocolate has more of these antioxidants than twenty-three different vegetables!

Dark chocolate is extremely concentrated with these polyphenols. Black tea is another good source of polyphenols. However, chocolate contains four times as much! You would have to eat 3.5 ounces of chocolate to obtain four times the amount of polyphenols in black tea. 3.5 ounces of chocolate is 525 calories! Tea has none. Sounds like a good reason to choose black tea, doesn't it?

Chocolate may have antioxidant benefits similar to vegetables but consider the numerous other benefits vegetables have that chocolate lacks. Vegetables provide fiber. Veggies also provide other disease fighting substances such as vitamins and minerals. Consider the caloric difference between an ounce of chocolate and one carrot. There is at least a 125-calorie difference and nine grams of fat!

Studies have yet to conclude whether chocolate's antioxidant health properties are as long lasting as that of vegetables. In one study, the benefits of chocolate's polyphenols diminished after only two hours. It takes months, even years of antioxidant presence in the blood to have an effect on your health. We do not know how much chocolate is necessary to produce this effect either.

Chocolate can be part of a healthy diet. It is acceptable to have a little chocolate now and then. Just don't eat it everyday.

67.

ORGANIC FOOD – IS IT WORTH IT?

You are probably familiar with the word "organic". But do you know what it means? The difference between organic and non-organic foods may leave many scratching their heads in confusion.

Organic food is an edible substance that is made possible without the use of pesticides or herbicides. Organic farming is a technique in which crops are rotated more often to nourish the soil. One year a farmer may plant tomatoes; the next year he'll plant green beans.

Organic food is safe for the environment. Pesticides, herbicides and fungicides can harm the food supply. It is a must to wash fresh produce before eating. Herbicides, pesticides, and fungicides eventually flow into Earth's natural water supply. Water then becomes toxic. Animals are harmed.

You probably knew animals could become extinct, but did you know the same is true for fruits and vegetables? There used to be approximately 300 varieties of carrots, only 21 remain! Similarly, there use to be 408 types of tomatoes. Now only 79 tomato species are left. Why? Conventional farming relies on seeds that make the produce ripen rapidly. Harvesting can be done much earlier, preventing seeds from naturally landing in the soil to reproduce. Wouldn't it be terrible if tomatoes became unavailable? You would have to eat pizza without the sauce!

You may think organic sounds healthy. It is healthy for nature; however there is not evidence that it is healthier for us. A few studies have been done and the results are mixed. There is not a significant enough difference between the vitamin and mineral content of organic produce and conventional produce to claim that one is healthier.

There is an obvious price difference. Organics usually range between 20-50 percent higher in cost. A regular large lemon will cost you about 60 cents; the organic lemon will cost you 90 cents. We have changed in the past decade. In 1997, General Mills was test-marketing an organic wheat flour that was to cost an entire dollar more that it's non-organic counterpart. Now organic grocers are popular. Organic food is continuously being advertised in popular magazines. The availability of organics in traditional grocers continues. The market must be there, which shows a nature-conscious world.

You are choosing organic food when you see the product displaying a logo from a third party certification agency. If the food label claims "organic" that means 95% of the ingredients within the product were organically produced. If a food product you see has the phrase "made with organic ingredients" on the label, this indicates that the main ingredients within the product are organic.

The American Dietetic Association promotes Earth conservation. The cost may be higher for organics but the land can be used for a longer duration. In the long run, this may be more cost-efficient and healthier for everyone.

68.

POUNDS WITH AGE... IS IT INEVITABLE?

Do you think that aging causes weight gain? Some think that it is out of our control. Your body is always changing. It did when you changed from a child to an adolescent. It will change when you become older as well. Hormones are reaching highs and lows, body structure grows, body chemistry is changing, and daily activities alter. Hormones that regulate metabolism tend to become less active as one ages. Most people lose bone and muscle tissue while gaining fat. Daily activity decreases. Your metabolism decreases when you do less. Therefore, your energy needs will decrease too. Either you have to eat less calories (energy) or you need to do more exercise if want to eat the same. Let's analyze a typical day for you:

At work:
Do you walk to destinations that are 2-3 blocks away?
Do you park far away from the building?
Does your occupation have you sitting or moving about?

Leisure Time Activities:
How many hours per week do you spend in your free time moving around?

Exercise:
How many hours per week do you exercise?

For example, Doris scored very low on all parts of this questionnaire other than for her exercise. She would rank as an inactive person if she didn't exercise. She sits in front of the computer for eight hours, sleeps for eight hours, dines for two hours, does housework for an hour, reads for a couple of hours, and works out for two hours. When you balance your activity level and eating as you age, you can keep your weight relatively steady.

Researchers have examined aging and weight gain more closely. Dr. Paul Williams took 5,000 runners between the ages of 18 and 49. He compared the running distances, weight gain, etc. A man would have to increase the length that he runs by 1.4 miles per week for every year of his life to prevent weight gain. That calculates to 14 extra miles a week after 10 years!

A nutrition expert will estimate a lower amount of calories for each year a person is old. For example, a woman weighing 125 pounds standing five foot six would need fifty calories less at age 30 as opposed to age 20. Scientific evidence shows that a metabolism will slow as one ages. It is unclear whether it is because of physiological changes or alterations in activity level.

You can do your own research. Test your body by trying to maintain its activity level. If you are sitting all day, take five hours a week for cardiovascular exercise. Add 2 hours a week of strength training. Do two more hours of stretching exercise such as yoga or Pilates. Take every chance you get to walk to destinations. Determine whether weight gain is inevitable with age!

69.

BODY BUILDERS WASTING MONEY

The health, fitness and nutrition market is enormous. There are phonies that sell nutritional and fitness products with no benefit. Believe it or not, you do not need supplements to build muscle. In fact, protein supplements can be harmful!

The best way to build muscle is through muscle enduring activities. That is opposite of what the phonies want you to think. In the early 1900's, supplements were not prevalent. Most people had labor-intensive jobs. Muscle building was inevitable. That is because they were doing muscle-enduring activities.

Protein supplements can be dangerous. Our bodies are not meant to receive such large quantities of protein. The kidney can fail from overdose of protein. The long-term risk of taking protein supplements far outweighs any short-term benefit!

When you take protein supplements, not all of the protein is digested. The traditional protein found in food is digested and absorbed much better.

Amino acids are a popular protein supplement. Some people choose to take one type of amino acid. However, when one amino acid is magnified in consumption, it minimizes the absorption of other amino acids possibly leading to malnourishment. The amino acid taken in abundance can promote toxicity. Just because a nutrient does good things in our body, does not mean more is better.

It is best to receive the benefits of protein the normal way – through eating a balanced diet with protein, carbohydrate and a little fat. It is a more economical and tasty way to obtain protein.

70.

EATING ON THE ROAD

When you are taking a road trip it can be so easy to eat out of boredom. The typical vacationing car packs a snack bag containing items such as chips, cookies, pretzels, snack mix, candy and dry cereal. You stop at a restaurant for lunch. You hop back into the car and there sitting beside you is a bag of chocolate chip cookies. Rid yourself of the temptation and take these helpful traveling snacking tips with you on your next journey.

Snacking – Nix the chips, snack mix, dry cereal, pretzels and hard candies. Once you start eating snacks like these you cannot stop. Bring chopped celery and carrots to munch on. You will be saving yourself at least 65 calories per handful. Pack a bag of apples, oranges or even dried fruit such as raisins.

Drinking – Fruit juices and milk are not liquids you want to be sipping on the duration of the trip. Drink lots of ice water. Add lemons, limes or orange slices for flavor. If you like soda, drink diet.

Chewing - Chew sugarless gum. Chewing gum actually helps your body burn more calories and it keeps your mouth busy so you don't want to constantly snack.

Restaurants - When dining out along the way, choose healthy entrees. If you must have fries, order a small and share them with someone. You can also take advantage of the low-fat/calorie options.

Just remember to pack light in terms of food. This will prevent you from taking extra pounds home as a souvenir.

71.

EATING OUT

Going out to eat is a real treat! It is a time to unwind in an atmosphere that suits our mood. Unfortunately, there is one major downfall to eating out. It's the damage it does to the waistline! A study done at the University of Memphis found that women who eat out six or more times per week consume an extra 300 calories per day. That calculates to twenty-four pounds per year!

Here is some advice to remember when dining out. Use the acronym "**LEAN**". This is everything you need to know.

"L" ight Menu - Most restaurants offer sensational tasting healthy choices. They add flavor without the fat and calories. Always choose from the light menu.

"E" njoy - Enjoy every substance you put into your mouth and savor it. Take the time to enjoy the first sip of crystal clear water served when you arrive to the last spoonful of sorbet. You will feel satisfaction from savoring the moment of every bite. Talk to your dining companion. This will help slow your eating pace and allow you to take pleasure in your food.

"A" sk - Ask your server questions about the food on the menu. For example, you are dining at a French restaurant and see the words "beurre blanc" with chicken. You know chicken would be a very healthy option but what is "beurre blanc"? If you ask the server, you will find out this peculiar word means white butter. Be assertive…ask!

"N" ix - Nix the appetizer and high calorie desserts! You will not enjoy your main entrée if you are already full. It is difficult to say "no" to dessert especially when the server shows you the dessert tray. Opt for a cappuccino made with skim milk, a frozen sorbet or a fruit cup.

You don't have to say "no" to eating out. Just remember the **"LEAN"** acronym to make smarter choices.

72.

KEEP GOING!

Being healthy can be difficult at times. Determination will help you reach your goals. This new way of life will get easier the longer you stay with it. You will actually like the taste of healthy foods. You will choose the healthy option without even thinking about it. You will appreciate an occasional small order of French fries but too many days in a row of this will make you feel unpleasant. You will feel pain each time you miss your workout. Believe it or not, you will be aching to take a jog, or whatever form of exercise is most desirable to you.

Keep going even in the face of cold opposition. Do not let anyone ever determine your life. You may experience ridicule when you decide to make the choice to change your lifestyle. Use this negative feedback to energize you! It's sometimes a great feeling to prove someone wrong. Instead, make sure you fill your life with positives. Optimist friends and family are a blessing. They are encouraging and want what is best for you. They are not envious and love you truly from their heart. Use this positive feedback to energize you as well.

Remember for healthy weight loss, losing one to two pounds per week is best. You want to lose it slowly in order to maintain it for the rest of your life. At times this may seem to take forever, but that calculates to 104 pounds per year. A year goes by pretty fast. Keep going!

73.

EVERY LITTLE BIT COUNTS

Do you know what matters when it comes to dieting? Even the croutons on your salad make a difference. A handful of chocolates in the middle of the day will keep you from meeting your goals. How about the Fourth of July? You are on vacation from work so might as well put the diet on vacation too, right?

Every little bit of eating counts. What makes you think that your body is not going to recognize that handful of chocolates as calories? Your body recognizes all food as energy. The unused energy is stored as fat. Many times we eat food out of habit instead of eating when we really need or want the food. The key to dieting is to change these unnecessary habits. Instead of making it a tradition to grab a handful of chocolates each time you pass through the mailroom, fill your hands with your mail only and head back to your desk. It is okay to treat yourself to one moderate handful of chocolate candies once a week. Save it for a time when you are really craving chocolate. The chocolate will be much more enjoyable.

During holidays many people vacation from eating in moderation. People think that gaining weight over the Holiday season is acceptable. Most people do not lose the weight gained over the Holiday. If they have this attitude next Holiday season, they'll add another five pounds! Food is abundant during other occasions too. This includes: Super bowl Sunday, Valentine's Day, Fat Tuesday, Passover, Mother's Day, Father's Day, wedding showers, birthday parties, family reunions, the Fourth of July, and on and on! You should not break from healthy eating. You can plan for these special days. Do this by budgeting your food intake. It's okay to have one cinnamon roll on Christmas morning. But forego the Christmas cookies on the table nearby.

Eating in moderation is about eating high-calorie foods when they fit into your food budget. Fill the rest of your day with whole grains, low-fat proteins, fruits, and last but definitely not least…vegetables!

74.

DON'T GO GROCERY SHOPPING WITHOUT ME

Do you go grocery shopping with good intentions and leave with a few more treats than you had planned? This is common. You may want to try grocery shopping by yourself. Mysteriously items appear in the cart when you bring other people like your kids and your spouse! It also helps to make a grocery list before you go. Only buy items from your list.

Produce – Sixty percent of your time should be spent in the produce aisle. Buy your snacks here. Choose ready-to-eat baby carrots, celery sticks, and broccoli florets. Make sure you grab leafy greens to make healthy salads. Choose a high nutrient green such as spinach or romaine. Anything and everything in this aisle are fabulous choices for healthy eating.

Dairy – One percent and fat-free milk have *all* the calcium and nutrients that whole milk has. They just have fewer saturated fat grams and calories. Soymilk is extremely healthy, tastes great and for lactose intolerant people contains *no* lactose! Make sure your soymilk is fortified with calcium. Pick up a large carton of fat free, sugar-free flavored yogurt. Select the low-fat cheeses over their regular counterparts. When opting for margarine, pick one that is lower in trans-fatty acids. Egg substitutes are significantly lower in calories and cholesterol than eggs.

Canned – Peanut butter is a nutritious way to make a quick lunch. Natural peanut butter is an excellent source of healthy fat and protein. As long as you can keep a jar of peanut butter in the kitchen without sticking a spoon into it every night, go ahead and grab a jar – crunchy or creamy - and use it in moderation. There are numerous canned foods to describe. Basically, your focus in this aisle should be to pick foods containing as little additives (saturated fat, sugar, salt) as possible and choose the ones with nutritional benefits (fiber, vitamins and minerals).

Bread & Cereal – Take advantage of all of the fiber in this aisle. Some of the cereals in this aisle can dramatically help you attain your goal of 20-35 grams of fiber per day. With one small serving of some wheat bran cereals you consume at least one-third of your recommended amount of fiber. Choose the whole wheat or whole grain bread. Sounds easy, right? Not so. Many shoppers are fooled. Check the ingredient labels of "wheat bread". The bread must read "whole wheat flour" as the first ingredient. This is necessary to receive the benefits of whole grain.

Meats– You'll know which cuts of meat are lean if you remember these: loin, round and flank. Select rib, chuck or rump for a roast. As for ground meat, choose the ones that are labeled as lean or very lean. A majority of your protein choices should consist of poultry and seafood with a few cuts of lean red meat. Because there are so many cuts of meat available, it is advised to read the food label carefully to compare fat content.

Try other delicious meat alternatives. Start with sampling a veggie burger. Vegetarian selections have health benefits and are high in cancer fighting anti-oxidants. These selections are also low in saturated fat. You can try soy cheeses, meat analogs such as tofu hot dogs, veggie breakfast sausage links and vegetarian "meat balls". The options are amazingly diverse!

Frozen – Br-r-r-r! Grab your coat for this aisle. Frozen vegetables are a great alternative to fresh vegetables and are a better choice than canned. If you like juice for breakfast, this is the most cost-effective place to look. Choose a juice without added sugar and choose a variety of juices such as orange, grapefruit and grape. You may even want to look for juices fortified with calcium for an extra boost. Stick to the lower fat entrees if you buy convenience meals. Check out the whole grain toaster waffles, pancakes and bagels. Choose frozen yogurt, sherbet, low fat ice cream or fruit juice bars for low fat dessert options.

Dry Goods – This is the moderation aisle! You should only consume these foods occasionally. Only buy the boxed mixes for special occasions. I recommend choosing whole-wheat flour and making pancakes from scratch rather than buying the pancake mix. Light syrup is a nice substitute for regular syrup. If you really want to be nutritious, top your pancakes with fresh fruit instead!

Drinks – Most of what you find in this aisle is none other than sugar. Try not to drink regular soda pop. Diet soda is a better option if you crave a carbonated beverage. If you like beer, go for light! It is half the calories. Wine can be another option. One glass of red wine with your dinner will have positive effects on the lipid levels in your blood. Be careful not to drink too much. It can increase your calories considerably.

Snacks – This is *not* the snack aisle. Remember? That was the first aisle we went down where we filled half our cart with produce. Look around you. Do you see anyone that is fit? The only snacks you should buy are pretzels, popcorn or baked chips. Get out before the fat demons find you!

Go to the check out counter. Congratulate yourself on your most cost-effective grocery trip ever. You will get the most bang-for-your-buck if you buy items that I recommended in this chapter. Paying for foods that have the greatest value inside the body is the mindset of a smart grocery shopper!

75.

CHILD INFLUENCE

We should teach children as early as possible the importance of good health, balanced nutrition and activity. According to recent reports and studies, American children are becoming more overweight. Some American children are even developing adult-onset diabetes (a disease attributed primarily to being overweight as an adult)! With the high technology video games, Internet and unsafe streets, it is no wonder kids are inactive.

Becoming overweight at such a young age has detrimental physical and social ramifications. Social isolation, rejection, and distorted body image are immediate consequences. As adults, these children experience higher risks for cardiovascular disease, diabetes, cancer and even disorders in sleep patterns.

Many children have nutritional habits we all should mimic. Healthy children eat by instinct. When they are hungry they eat and when they are not hungry they do not eat. That is why experts debate the practice of making children clean their plate before leaving the table. Somehow as adults we learn to eat by external cues, ignoring our inner cues. We eat more because the server brought by the dessert tray and we couldn't resist the temptation even though we were miserably full. We eat less because we saw an attractive model on television that must starve to achieve that look but we want to look that way. We need to teach children to hold onto this instinct they have. By not making them clean their plates is one way to assist children in developing health-eating habits. Make them realize that everyone's body is different.

Do not force food on children. For example, if little Billy is not eating his entire dinner, do not force him to eat. However, if Billy is hungry one hour later for potato chips, his dinner should be brought back out as opposed to the potato chips he desires.

It can be challenging to help children make nutritious choices at an early age. This is because of their amazing sweet tooth. Children choose sweet foods in greater quantities when they think no one is watching. Some sugar is okay. Explain to the child what happens when they have too much sugar such as painful cavities. Sugar can make some foods more appealing to children. You can give your child vegetables by smearing peanut butter on celery stalks.

Children need to learn to be active. This can be challenging. Sugar intake is not a concern when a child is active. Encourage the child to play outside, become involved in extra-curricular activities and participate willingly in gym class. Demonstrate to the child that it is "cool" to be active. Be a good example yourself. Walk to the store when it is only one block down the road and exercise on a regular basis. You are your child's best influence.

76.

DROP POUNDS, SAVE MONEY, EAT THE SAME

How would you like to lose pounds *and* save money? You could use the savings to buy new clothes in a slimmer size. Wouldn't it be nice if you didn't have to change the way you eat? I'm assuming the answer is yes.

There is only one catch. You must currently consume high calorie beverages such as regular soda pop, creamed and sugared coffee, sweetened fruit drinks, beer or sweetened tea. Most of us do.

The calories you drink in a day can really add up. You will save 1050 calories per week by eliminating one of these beverages per day. You will lose 1.2 pounds if you do this for a month! That's 14.4 pounds a year and several hundred dollars!

This can be difficult. Soda pop compliments pizza so nicely. Sweetened tea is delightful on a hot summer day. Lemonade tastes better than plain water. A morning without coffee is like summer without sun. And there is nothing like a tasty beer at 5 p.m. on Friday. Try drinking water more often. There are other beverages besides water that you can choose. The secret is to drink zero calorie beverages ninety percent of the time. Diet soda pop tastes better once you acquire a taste for it. Tea drinkers can add flavor to their tea with lemons or artificial sweetener. If you like coffee, drink it black. Is this too strong? Use artificial sweetener and a bit of skim milk. Drink beer occasionally - once or twice a week. You can save up to 55 calories per can if you choose light instead of regular.

Scott entered college and decided to drink diet soda instead of regular. He also gave up snacking. Scott lost forty pounds by the end of his first semester. Small adjustments in your lifestyle can lead to big changes. Drinking low calorie beverages is perhaps the easiest change you'll make.

77.

LESS CALORIES, MORE FILLING

Eating foods and beverages with air incorporated into them will help you lose weight. Research indicates that people who eat this type of food actually consume fewer calories throughout the entire day.

Though you cannot see it or feel it, air takes up space. Think of a balloon. It gets bigger by blowing air into it. If you blow too much air into a balloon it pops. If your stomach is full of air, you feel full. Eating more makes you feel uncomfortable. The air that makes you full is calorie free.

So what kind of air can satisfy your hunger? There are several delicious food and beverage items full of air. You may cringe when you spend six dollars at the movie theater for a tub of popcorn, which is predominately air.

Eat puffed rice or puffed wheat in a bowl topped with skim milk and fruit for breakfast. Pack a crispy rice treat or rice cake for your lunch dessert. While you dine, sip on sparkling water flavored with lemon.

Calorie-free stomach filler is water. Drink water all day to keep your belly full. Crisp fruit and refreshing vegetables are 95 percent water. Even meats and cheeses are 50 percent water but are not very low in calories and fat. You should eat bountiful amounts of fruits and vegetables everyday. These hydrated stomach-filling food items taste great and provide the body with vitamins, minerals and fiber!

Air and water are two essential ingredients for life. You are bound to end up with fewer calories when you incorporate them into every meal.

78.

AGING WITH GRACE

Do you think age prevents you from staying in shape? Would you like to be fit and healthy at age eighty? It's possible!

My grandma is an extraordinary role model for all of us. She discovered her passion for golf during her twenties. She perfected her game by playing four times per week and progressed to the top of her league. There are two amazing "hole-in-one" pictures of her at the country club in Iron River, Michigan. She has won several tournaments in her golf career. Perhaps the best trophy she has won is the healthy body she still maintains. At age eighty-one, she plays the game several times per week.

Are you afraid you cannot find a lifetime activity to enjoy? You must be persistent. There is something for everyone. This activity does not have to be a sport. Dancing is my passion. Some people view dancing as an art but it's also an extreme exercise. Once you find an activity that you enjoy, practice it frequently. Set your goals high and motivate yourself to become better. It is incredibly rewarding to become exceptional at a skill.

The pressure to maintain a healthy weight increases when you mature. Active adults do not feel this burden. The metabolism typically decreases with age. Being active increases it. This allows active adults to eat a well balanced diet.

Active adults are also more in tune with their appestat. The appestat is the part of the hypothalamus that regulates hunger level. This allows these individuals to eat when they are truly hungry.

79.

CHOOSE GREEN DRINKS

Green drinks represent a category of drinks rather than a color. Not all beverages are created equal in terms of being good choices for drinking often. There are three-color categories for drinks. Green drinks are the ones you drink most often, red drinks are occasional drinks and yellow drinks are somewhere in between.

One of the keys to maintaining a healthy weight and being optimally healthy is drinking a plethora of liquids, especially the big one – *water!* No other drink is as safe as water when drinking it in large quantities. Carry water with you all day to keep yourself hydrated and full. Try to carry a 32 oz. water bottle with you everywhere you go. Always have water at restaurants. Alternate between your ordered drink and water. Don't confine yourself to only water served ice cold. Order a mug of hot water with a lemon wedge. This is a great drink when it's cold outside!

Drink tap water once in a while because it contains fluoride. Some bottled water is not fluorinated. Water definitely belongs to the green category.

There are liquids deserving a yellow category meaning caution or in daily moderation. Drinks that are healthy are not necessarily drinks that you consume in vast quantities. Fruit juice is a good example. I had one client who eliminated her gestational diabetes by limiting her fruit juice intake to no more than 1-cup per day. Skim and 1% milk are other yellow category drinks. Drink two to three glasses per day for strong bones.

Alcohol is another yellow category drink. Drink one drink per day for heart health. If you drink alcohol, it is desirable to do so in moderation drinking one to ten drinks per week. The yellow category alcohol drinks are

4 oz. wine (red or white) or a 12 oz. light beer. Dark beer has heart health benefits similar to wine however it is not as low in calories as light beer.

There are some yellow drinks called free-drinks. These are drinks that are calorie-free, such as diet soft drinks. However these drinks should not be abused or consumed in large quantities. Once a day is fine but don't let them replace your water intake.

You can have red category drinks occasionally. Some examples of red drinks are: Margaritas, Long Island Ice Teas, Pina Coladas, Daiquiris, 2% and higher percent fat milk, sodas, fruit drinks, milk shakes, large sugary smoothies, and sugared coffee drinks. If you are drinking mostly red drinks, try switching to green or calorie-free yellow drinks. I guarantee you'll lose weight.

80.

CONTROLLING YOUR BLOOD SUGAR

Do you wonder why you feel weak and tired at about 4 p.m.? If you experience weakness, dizziness, fatigue, irritability, sweatiness, confusion, blurred vision, shakiness, palpitations, anger, and/or headaches you are a probable candidate for hypoglycemia.

Here is a typical scenario. Monet is a busy twenty-year-old female. She spends twenty hours a week in dance class, not to mention the extra hours she spends practicing on her own.

Monet had a warm zucchini nut muffin with a pat of margarine one day for breakfast. She had to make a quick trip to the drug store. When she walked back to her car, she started to feel very weak, irritable and shaky.

Monet has a fast metabolism because of her high activity level. The one muffin she ate in the morning wasn't enough to last until lunchtime. When she ate the muffin, the calories from it were absorbed into her bloodstream. The cells absorbed all of the energy and left the blood with little. And this is why Monet was weak because her blood was low on energy. This is known as, "low blood sugar". You may have also heard of hypoglycemia. Hypo means "low" and glycemia is "sugar".

If you experience the symptoms I described, you need to supply your blood with energy by eating immediately. Low blood sugar can occur for several reasons. This includes not eating enough food; missing a meal or snack, exercise without refueling the body with energy and/or having alcohol. Carry a snack around with you at all times. A convenient one would be trail mix. The mixture of carbohydrate in the raisins and fat and protein in the nuts is the perfect combination for sustained energy release.

The key is to feed your body when it is hungry. If you're to the point where you are shaking and irritable, a snack such as fruit juice will help you feel better. You need quick absorbing energy.

Developing communication between your body and brain is important for adequate functioning. Don't ignore hunger signals, especially when they get to the point as I have explained. Even if you are dieting, choose a light snack, one that coincides with your diet. Healthy eating includes small snacks throughout the day. One of the best ways to eat is 4 to 6 small meals per day.

81.

EATING FOR CANCER PREVENTION

Cancer is a health epidemic that is unfortunately too common. Everyone knows someone who has had cancer. It is in our best interest to prevent it from happening.

One major way you can decrease your risk of cancer is to maintain a healthy weight. Losing weight is not merely for appearance.

> **Case study** - The calorie consumption was restricted on obese laboratory rats. Their cancer risk decreased significantly.

Why do obese people have a higher risk for cancer? The extra fat traps carcinogens that one-day could develop into cancer. Another reason is that obese people typically do not eat enough healthy disease fighting foods such as fruits and vegetables.

Fat gets a bad rap for being the culprit of many health problems, including cancer. People that over consume fat and consume the wrong types of fat are the ones at risk. Omega 3 is an unsaturated type of fat that has been shown to prevent cancer. Omega 3's can be found in fish such as mackerel, salmon and herring. Eating Omega 6 Fatty Acid in large quantities promotes cancer. Omega 6 is found in vegetable oil. Use olive or canola oil instead. Beware of saturated and trans-fatty acids also.

Aim for 20 to 35 grams of fiber everyday for ultimate cancer prevention. Fiber is not digested and it traps carcinogens from being absorbed by the body. Fiber can be found in all types of fruits, vegetables, legumes and whole grains. These foods also contain invaluable phytochemicals. Phytochemicals help your immune system fight cancer.

Studies show that women who obtain Vitamin D from food decrease their risk of breast cancer by thirty percent. Milk is a wonderful source of vitamin D.

Be sure to eat a diet low in salt-cured, pickled or smoked foods. If you must drink alcohol, do so in moderation. If cancer is in your family history, you should restrict yourself to no more than one glass for women and two glasses for men. One drink is equivalent to the following:

> 12 oz. Wine Cooler
> 1 ½ oz. Liquor
> 5 oz. Wine
> 3 oz. Sherry or Port
> 12 oz. Regular or Light Beer

These cancer-preventing guidelines are similar to tips that ward off other diseases. That goes to show that eating healthy has a wide array of benefits.

82.

GET YOUR ZZZZZZ'S!

The average human needs between eight and ten hours of shut eye a night. There are very few people who can survive on only six hours. Proper sleep is very beneficial when it comes to overall wellness. Sleep can assist in the battle of weight loss along with many other health benefits. Studies show that your body metabolizes fat better with proper sleep.

Another health benefit related to sleep is that your brain will function optimally. When you are tired, you do not make wise choices. Thus your food choices may not be ideal either. Some people even eat to keep awake!

The immune system performs better with adequate sleep. Staying healthy will enable you to miss less work, keep up with your workouts and be active! All three of those measures burn more calories than lying in bed suffering from a cold with twenty-four hour access to a freezer stocked with fattening ice cream!

Sleep deprivation contributes to being grumpy, pessimistic, and having a nonchalant attitude. Without sleep, where are you going to get the will power to eat only one of your mother's homemade chocolate chip cookies? How are you going to convince yourself to go to the gym instead of going home to watch television? In a challenging situation, such as weight loss, you need will power. This comes with sleep.

83.

EMOTIONAL EATING

When you are stressed, what is your emotional release? People have different ways of handling emotion. Some deal with emotion positively while others deal negatively. Eating is a negative emotional outlet. Some people eat food when feeling blue, bored, or even bliss. All of us are confronted with several emotions every day. Eating due to emotional changes can cause weight gain.

Think about last week and the emotions you encountered. Did you eat food in order to deal with any of the emotions? If yes, did you feel better, did you feel worse or did your feelings not change at all?

> **1st Case Study** - Female A had a terrible day. She made herself a healthy chicken stir-fry dinner. Female A skipped working out because she was in a bad mood. She watched the beautiful actresses on her favorite television show. She felt guilty because she missed her workout. She drove to the nearest burger joint and ordered a burger, large fries, large cola and chicken tenders to go. After she ate, she went to bed even more depressed.

This is an example of emotional eating. Notice the snowball effect. When she first arrived home she only had a terrible day to deal with. As the night went on she compounded the problem by missing her workout and eating twice. She should have exercised the way she planned. The exercise would have elevated her mood. If you have a bad day, do not use this as an excuse to skip your workout. During physical activity your body releases a chemical called, "serotonin" to the brain. Serotonin triggers an uplifting feeling. Here are some other ways to deal with emotion:

- Sing or play a musical instrument

- Talk to a positive friend

- Turn on the radio and dance

- Play with your pet

- Meditate or do yoga

- Clean the house

- Work in the garden

- Play a video game

- Paint, draw or do other crafty activities

- Journal

- Surf the internet

Some people also eat during happy times. Perhaps one feels as if he or she deserves a treat for feeling good. Do not destroy the mood by pigging out and feeling guilty later on. Choose wisely when eating at joyous occasions.

2nd Case Study - Female B celebrated with her girlfriends by having a party. Her friends and she enjoy eating however all of them are unhappy with their weight. Female B stocked up on bags of chips and dip, gallons of ice cream, ordered four pizzas and cheesy breadsticks among other fun foods. The girls had a great night together but the next morning each one felt guilty for eating so much. Some of the girls left feeling irritable. This caused Female B to feel sad.

Food is a fun item to have during one of these celebrations. However Female B could have prevented the "I'm so fat" morning-after feeling by choosing low-fat munchies. Here is a list of foods that are fabulous food ideas to snack on for happy occasions:

- Raw veggies with low-fat dip

- Fresh fruit with yogurt dip

- Shrimp with cocktail sauce

- Air-popped popcorn with fat-free margarine sprayed on top

- Frozen yogurt or low-fat ice cream (no added sugar type) with fruit topping

- Baked chips with refried beans and fat-free sour cream dip

- Thin crust pizza with cheese and veggies

Consider talking to a counselor who can help you handle your emotions positively. Consulting with an expert can be a wise choice when battling life's struggles.

84.

HANDLING HEALTHY EATING WHEN VISITING OTHERS

Healthy eating can be tricky when you visit your friends and family. It is especially difficult when you go to visit a loved one and they have foods made for you that are calorie and fat laden. When you walk into their place you face bars, nuts, beer and chips and on top of all this they have plans to go out for dinner! Dinner is going to be the local steak house and the ice cream shop is planned for after dinner delights. How can you get through this without putting on all the weight you lost? People can become very offended when you do not partake of their food.

In most cases when visiting distant friends or relatives, the polite host provides an opportunity for you to offer a suggestion in event planning. Be sure to take them up on this offer! This is your chance to provide some ideas of "healthy" activities you would like to engage in. Do not limit your thinking to only food activities. Ask your host if there are beautiful hiking trails nearby that you could try biking, walking or roller-blading on. Make suggestions that would allow you to manage your diet, like Asian food. This type of food most often is lower in fat and calories than Mexican, Italian or American cuisine. Your host may want to know what kind of food you like. Suggest a few healthy dishes. Offer to help make dinner, this way you can have control of the amount of added fat and other extra calories.

Suppose your host does not ask for your suggestions. According to etiquette books, you are the visitor and you still have the right to make suggestions concerning activities you would like to participate in. Timing is everything when offering your suggestions however! Perhaps an appropriate time would be when discussing events for the weekend. Make a casual suggestion such as, "I would enjoy dining at a vegetarian restaurant one night. Is there one that you know of in your area?" You have the right to make these suggestions being that you are the one spending the time and money to make the trip.

You cannot expect people you are visiting to want to do *everything* you suggest. In fact, it is actually mentally healthy, according to Emily Post's book on etiquette, that you and your host have "breathing space". Take time away from each other to make the trip more enjoyable. There is nothing wrong with you making it clear to your host, "I'm going to be taking a jog every morning at 7 a.m. Do you have any suggestions of a good place for me to jog?" This will give your host a chance to break from entertaining.

Another way to give your host a break, and cater to your own nutritional needs, is to treat yourself to dinner. Perhaps you enjoy a cuisine that is unusual or of different interest than your host. A vegetarian restaurant would be a suitable example in this case. You could say, "Jon and I are hoping to try a popular vegetarian restaurant while in the area. We thought Thursday would be a good night for us to do that. Do not worry about having to entertain us that night." In this case you could invite your host as a treat to them. You may want to leave it open for your host to choose whether or not they will join you. But clearly state that your feelings will not be hurt if they choose to stay home and relax for a bit. Extending the invite is entirely up to you. Regardless, you will have an opportunity to continue on with your nutritional focus at a restaurant of your choice.

Do you feel that there will not be much flexibility in your upcoming trip? I recommend you stay at a hotel. This will allow you to eat breakfast and lunch on your own time and exercise in between. You cannot be invited into a person's house and expect them to have cuisine fit exactly to your taste. I have witnessed situations with vegetarians visiting people and making it quite an uncomfortable event. I do not recommend changing your food beliefs if they are important. If you can budge just for the night, that would be optimal. Ask for a smaller piece of chicken or eat only half. For calorie watchers, choose the smallest dessert and leave some bites.

Travel the world, and while doing so visit friends and family. It is amazing how enhanced your relationship with others can be when you take the time to visit their grounds. People often gain weight when they travel. Traveling is not the culprit, you are ultimately the one making choices. Make sure you do not offend anyone. You want to enrich relationships not eliminate them!

85.

DISEASES ARE RACIAL

No matter what your race is, you are more susceptible to some diseases. Your genes in your race and your culture make you prone to certain health problems. Here are the diseases that each race should be concerned with.

African-Americans – This race deems a higher percentage of victims killed from heart disease than other races. Diabetes is also common. African-Americans risk hypertension. People suffering with both of these diseases also are susceptible to kidney disease. Studies show that cancer is frequent. The cancers to be most aware of are colon and rectal cancer and lung and bronchus cancer.

American Indians – Heart disease is frequently found in this ethnic group. Sixty-two percent of American Indians have risk factors for heart disease according to the Behavior Risk Factor Surveillance System 1997. Lung cancer is the most common form of cancer. The chances of being diabetic are 2.8 times higher than any other race.

Asian Americans – This race tends to have a lower risk of cancer. The cancers found most commonly are of the stomach and liver. Asian women are prone to osteoporosis.

Caucasian Americans – It is estimated that one out of every two Caucasian women will experience a bone fracture attributed to osteoporosis. Some Caucasian women are more likely to have anemia. Caucasian men are prone to cancer in the reproductive organs.

Hispanic Americans – Cardiovascular disease among women is common. Diabetes is also frequent in this race. Cervical and prostate cancers are diagnosed more often. Other cancers are less likely.

You are *not* exempt from any disease because of your race. Diseases are also genetic. Review your family history. What diseases are prevalent there? You are prone to these diseases also.

It is important to know what you need to avoid! Nutrition is a preventive medicine that is very effective. It is never too late to start. Celebrate today because you're preventing yourself from diseases tomorrow!

86.

OBSERVING YOUR RELIGION

Religion often involves food. Whether it is communion or fasting, rules or rituals, religious traditions are a part of many lives. Why do people use food in religion? There are various reasons. The fasting ritual may help prove one's devotion to God. Another person may feel fasting helps her to focus better on God. Whatever the reason, fasting isn't easy to do.

Some religions abstain from certain foods. Catholics eat fish on Fridays during Lent. It can be difficult to give up something in your diet. Nutrition experts will tell you not to eliminate foods from your diet. They will also tell you not to skip meals. So what is more important - your religion or your health?

For example, let's say your religion does not allow you to eat during daylight. In this case, weight loss can be very difficult. This is because you are extremely hungry at night. You will have the tendency to eat more than you should. The trick to fasting between dawn and dusk is to eat a well-balanced meal at dawn. A meal consisting of protein, fat, and carbohydrate is a good example. A meal containing a fair amount of fiber is another plus. Fiber takes longer to digest therefore you do not get hungry as quickly.

Here are some examples of healthy before-dawn fasting meals,

- Whole-wheat breakfast burrito with eggs, low-fat cheese, salsa, and beans

- Whole-wheat bagel with low-fat cream cheese and fruit on top

- Oatmeal with nuts sprinkled on and a touch of vanilla extract

- Whole-wheat pancakes spread with peanut butter

When dinnertime finally arrives, take a deep breath and relax. Tell yourself, "not to overdo it." Start with a glass of water then a broth soup. This will wake up your insides and prepare you for digestion. Eat a balanced meal that includes lean protein. Add a carbohydrate high in fiber (whole wheat spaghetti or brown rice), green salad with light dressing, and cooked veggies drizzled with olive oil. Have frozen yogurt for dessert if you desire.

It is also difficult to exercise when you fast. You will feel very weak. If you can't exercise during the day, take a nice quick walk after finishing your evening meal. Find a companion to walk with you.

Another religion may require you to abstain from certain foods. When tempted by foods you are abstaining from:

- Relax, take a deep breath

- Drink a tall glass of water.

- Remind yourself it is well worth it.

So much of our world is filled with food. Food seems to be a focus at social gatherings, cultural events, and holidays. It's no surprise that food also shows up in our religions.

87

IS IT SODA OR IS IT POP?

To accommodate all regions of America let's call it "soda pop". How much or how little of this beverage should you drink? The USDA Food Guide Pyramid places soda pop at the top of the pyramid. The guideline says, "Drink sparingly." Those of you who prefer an exact number may want to know how much sparingly is.

The role soda pop plays in a person's diet is important. Is soda pop replacing nutrient-rich beverages? This is of special concern for growing children and adolescents. Drinking soda pop instead of calcium rich beverages inhibits calcium from entering the body. Children and adolescents need two to four cups of calcium rich drinks per day.

Soda pop is packed with sugar. That is where all of its calories are derived from. Sugar is "empty calories". Empty calories are calories with no nutrients other than energy. Drinking unlimited amounts of soda promotes obesity.

Diet sodas are calorie free. They are sweetened with aspartame, which is a non-nutritive sweetener. There is quite a lot of controversy regarding aspartame. Is aspartame cancerous or not? Thus far, aspartame shows not to be cancerous; therefore the FDA has approved it as an allowed additive to foods and beverages. Aspartame has not been around long enough to determine the long-term affects.

Soda pop is an acidic beverage. This can be harmful to the stomach, especially for people with ulcers. Too much soda pop makes for extensive acidic contact with the enamel on the teeth. This may promote erosion of the enamel. Try to drink soda pop through a straw most of the time.

Soda pop is the morning beverage of choice for some people who do not drink coffee. For those people, soda pop tastes better than coffee.

There are positive and negatives to caffeine. Some people suggest soda pop can cause acne. However this has not been proven.

There is only one answer...drink sparingly! Sparingly is no more than one a day- even the calorie free sodas. Drink water instead. You can also drink carbonated water; also known as unflavored seltzer water. Add fruit wedges to spice it up. Whether you drink soda or you drink pop, be sure to drink it sparingly.

88.

WORKING OUT WITH WEIGHTS

Weightlifting is the exercise of exhausting the muscles through repetitions of moving a load greater than what the muscle is use to. Weightlifting has increased in popularity, especially with women. Weightlifting is a must if you want a way to lose or maintain weight. It has a phenomenal effect on you metabolism. Muscle burns calories at a faster rate than fat. That's not the only perk; it builds strong bones and prevents fragility.

Choose eight exercises to work eight different muscle groups. This will yield more than an hour workout. First, you must warm your muscles with a light cardiovascular activity such as walking, jogging, stair climbing or bicycling. It is important to set the weightlifting machines in the appropriate position for your body size. Improper alignment can cause injury. This is becoming more common as people lift weights carelessly.

It is a good idea to choose opposing muscle groups. An example of opposing muscle groups is the biceps and the triceps. Otherwise one muscle becomes too strong while the other one stays weak. The other muscle groups you should work out are: deltoids (shoulder muscles), abdominal muscles, back muscles, hamstrings, quadriceps, and gluteus maximums.

Weightlifting is best if done 2-3 days per week with one day of rest between lifting days. For example, you can lift weights on Monday, Wednesday and Friday. This leaves Tuesday, Thursday, and Saturday for cardiovascular exercising. Finally you can rest on Sunday.

There are many options for weightlifting workout plans. The most common plan is three sets of ten repetitions. Go with fewer sets if you do not want to be "too big". For those of you worried about becoming "too big" I recommend you go with fewer sets more repetitions. For serious muscle builders, start off with a moderate weight doing 12 repetitions. For the next set, decrease the weight slightly and move down to 10 repetitions. Continue this decreasing of weight until you do two more sets of 8 and 6.

When weightlifting, do not go into autopilot and begin lifting carelessly. Think about what you are doing. Weightlifters who concentrate on their muscles while working out involve more muscle fibers. Your chances of injury are less also. Don't do the repetitions too fast. You'll engage more muscle fibers if you do the movements slowly. Take about four seconds for the lift, and four seconds for the release. Never lift alone. This is another way to be injured.

Take an opportunity to lengthen and stretch the muscles you have been contracting and shortening. The more you can lengthen a muscle, the further it can contract. This builds more strength. Moderate stretching also prevents injuries from occurring in the future. Stretch for at least five minutes during your workout.

There is no reason to change your diet because you have added weightlifting to your routine. Eat a balanced diet. The only lifters who need to alter their diet are the world-class competitive lifters who lift more than three times a week. If you are one of those, you need to add more protein to your diet. This is to rebuild the muscle that you tear from lifting.

Add a new aspect to your workout if begins to get boring. You can choose new muscle groups to work on. Buy an exercise magazine for innovative workout routines.

You will become stronger in body and mind!

89.

Q.A. BY A R.D.

A Registered Dietitian – R.D. - has valid credentials and authority on nutrition. Quality Assurance – Q.A. – refers to making sure that the condition of an item, person or service is performing well. For example, a food critic that rates *quality* of service at a restaurant is providing Q.A. for the restaurant's owner.

How is your nutritional Q.A.? Quality Assurance is important to health. It may be the answer to your nutritional problems. It will be difficult to analyze your own health. I recently read a study sponsored by the National Cancer Institute. The focus of this study was to design a Quality Assurance program for nutrition data collection. Nutrition data collection refers to the measurement of amounts of food eaten. The margin of error in nutritional data collection is amazingly large. Consequently, this is why so many people do not lose weight when they diet. The study used two groups. Registered Dietitians used different data collection methods for each group. The Group A participants followed a diet and were called upon by the Registered Dietitians to report what had been eaten. The margin of error was low for this method of data collection. Group B reported all food eaten using diaries. This self-reporting method proved not to be as effective as the previous method.

Have you ever tried a weight-loss plan that wasn't effective? You should lose weight as long as you follow the plan. In these circumstances I recommend trouble-shooting the plan to see where the errors are arising. You could be counting 8 ounces of wine as one serving of alcohol instead of two. You could be recording French fries as a vegetable instead of a starch and a fat. These little errors go unnoticed. A Registered Dietitian can help you prevent errors that keep you from meeting your goal.

It is important to get a nutrition check-up annually. A Registered Dietitian will judge your eating style more objectively. Perhaps you need an expert to analyze your judgment of portion sizes. Not understanding portion sizes can attribute to undesirable plateau periods during the process of weight loss. It may cost a little time and money but it may also be the answer to your nutritional dilemma!

90.

LOVIN' THOSE HANDLES

Do you have a spare tire around your middle? Last time you were at a wedding, did this happen to you: you were choo-chooing with a long train of people around the dance floor to the catchy tune, "Come On Ride the Train," and the person behind you had no problem hanging on. Your spare tire around the middle was way too easy to hold on to. Or, the last time you hugged your sarcastic younger sister did she grab the sides of you and exclaim, "Boy, you got a lot of lovin here!" Ouch, painful thoughts but oh so true. The good news is there is hope!

That spare layer of fat around your middle does not need to stay with you for the rest of your life. Good heavens, no! Take it off! Of course it's not as simple as taking off an article of clothing (well, not including those jeans that are way too tight). The answer to shedding that spare tire around the middle is not what you think it may be. It doesn't come off with tens of thousands of sit-ups or abdominal crunches and rollers. Taking off this fat involves two main ingredients in your life:

A diet high in vegetables

Aerobic activity most days of the week

Consider this study. Researchers at Washington University took a group of 60 to 70 year old men and women. Their lifestyle was changed from being sedentary to walking briskly or running for 45 minutes four times a week. These study subjects lost an average of one and a quarter inches around their middle in a little less than a year's time.

Not only were these people smiling at the thought of losing an inch around the middle, but their doctors were smiling also. Why? Because not only did they lose an inch around their waist, they also decreased their high cholesterol readings. Total blood cholesterol readings fell from an average of 205 milligrams/deciliter (mg/dL) to an average of 194 mg/dL. (Anything over 200 is considered high). Other measurements that also decreased were triglyceride levels (increases risk for heart disease) and blood sugar levels (depicting possible diabetes). As you can see, the advantages to shedding that layer of fat around your middle is good for your internal health as well as your physical image.

Now let's focus on what changes you need to make in your diet. A study performed by the American Cancer Society points to an eating style that includes lots of fresh vegetables to ward of abdominal fat. Researchers followed 80,000 people for ten years. In their research, those who ate nineteen servings of vegetables or more throughout the week were less likely to develop a layer of fat around their middle than those who ate very few vegetables. Additionally, those subjects who ate red meat three or more times per week were more likely to develop a band of fat around their waistline. "Why vegetables?" you ask. Scientists are not sure if it's a special mechanism inside vegetables that triggers fat burning or if those people just lead all-around healthier lifestyles. Either way, one thing is for sure…EAT YOUR VEGGIES!

If you are thinking, "Aahh, big deal! So I have an extra cushion around the middle. I'm not hurting anyone." Well, think again because you are hurting *yourself*. It is a fact that people who store fat around the abdominal region are at a much higher risk for heart disease than those who store fat around the hip area. This may sound familiar to you. We refer to people who store fat around the abdominal area as having an "apple shape". Those who store fat around the legs and buttocks are referred to as having a "pear shape". Although carrying only the amount of fat that is necessary for life is ideal, being pear shaped is preferred. More often men tend to be the apple shape and women the pear shape, although not always.

Though we are fooled by all of the abdominal machines on the market, they are not the answer to losing your gut. The answer lies right out your front door. Open the door, walk or run for an hour most days of the week.

Be faithful to this every week, and your gut will start to disappear. Don't neglect your diet either. You're not getting off that easy! You must watch your diet. Eat a diet plentiful in fresh vegetables. Instead of centering meals on meat entrees, try making vegetables the star of the meal. Now your tummy is really going to start to fade away. Good riddance!

91

PSYCHOLOGY OF ERGOGENIC AIDS

Many people use performance enhancing substances for maximum results. You may be surprised to find out how many people rely on ergogenic aids. Firefighters use these to enhance their performance in their job, professional athletes improve their homerun record, and coaches push young athletes into taking them.

Before my experience teaching nutrition to the fire departments, I was against taking these substances. However, I can understand why individuals would want to. Ergogenic aids provide increased ability to perform in lifting heavy objects. They also help with the pressures to "look good."

Sure the advantages of these popular substances are very tempting. However, I can't see the benefits outweighing the potential negative side effects. Negative side effects include: dehydration, taxing the kidney, personality changes, addiction, abuse, and improper measurement in administration, and even more.

What about the psychological aspects of ergogenic aids? For example, the athlete taking ergogenic aids to hit the ball out of the ballpark. The immediate benefits are overly tempting: fame and fortune. What is most important is that the athlete feels good about his health in the long run. How fulfilling is it knowing you reached your goal because you included foreign substances in the body? It is much more rewarding to obtain goals through hard work and determination.

Consider two athletes equally talented and tied in what they are competing for. Let us use two baseball players striving for the record-breaking homerun as an example. The first athlete, let's call him Rocky, has reached his level of play because of his disciplined training. The other athlete, let's name him Jake, reached his goal by hard work *and* ergogenic aid use. Who is the true champion? Rocky feels a deeper sense of accomplishment. How embarrassed Jake will feel when his miracle supplement is banned from his sport. We will witness the athlete's performance level gradually decline. Rocky will not be affected. His level of championship athleticism continues.

For those people relying on supplements for weight loss, consider these thoughts. Where is your sense of gratification going to come from? You will feel better if you conquer this challenge by disciplining yourself as opposed to popping a pill. If you are taking a supplement without exercise, your body may be thin, but will it be toned? A weight loss supplement will not increase your HDL levels. Your HDL levels benefit when you engage in physical activity.

Before ingesting any substance into your body, thoroughly weigh the pros and cons of short-term and long-term effects. Yes, it may be impressive to hit fifty homeruns in a baseball season but having your kidney fail early in life is not impressive!

92.

TALKING TO YOURSELF

Do you talk to yourself? Be honest! It's nothing to be ashamed of. We all do it! This self-talk can either be a good activity or extremely destructive. You can make it what you want. Positive talk can improve your health. Likewise, negative self-talk will do damage resulting in feelings of depression, anger and guilt.

You'll see results in your nutrition and fitness when you talk to yourself positively. You will lose weight easier and faster when you fill your mind with positive thoughts. You can buy a motivational book that will give you a quick positive thought to dwell on everyday.

Stop and think when you start to fret. Can you change the problem you are worrying about? It is changeable if the problem resides in you. Don't beat yourself up over the problem. Try to feel thankful that you realize a change needs to be made and make that change! If the problem resides in another individual, realize that this is out of your control. Use your time and energy for something more useful to you! Here are some positive things you can do:

- Do yoga!

- Surround yourself with positive people.

- Journal your thoughts and feelings.

- Love yourself.

- Seek positive affirmation from only yourself.

- Believe that good things will happen to you.

- Be proud of whom you are and the changes you are making!

It is challenging to think positively all the time, especially when people around you are feeling negative. Keep your interaction with these people to a minimum. Many times these negative attitudes can affect our own lives. You can't change the way they behave. You're going to have to change yourself instead.

Prepare to shrug at negative comments when around these people. Do not let it get to you. Don't fight back, don't give a look, just be the strong one. Know in your heart that you are thinking positively about yourself, life and the world! Usually the one being negative to you ends up looking foolish to those around you.

Begin your positive self talk today! Be patient with yourself. It is worth it no matter how long it takes you.

93

STOPPING WORLD HUNGER

You probably have donated in some way to the problem of world hunger. Maybe you contributed or walked/ran a 5K race. You may have attended a fund raising concert that aided hunger in Africa. There's another way to help decrease world hunger. It's eating less animal meat.

The world is dependent upon the efficiency of its food chain. The food chain looks similar to the food-guide pyramid. It is represented as a triangle with three tiers. It represents the flow of food in our ecological system.

At the bottom of the triangle are the vegetarian entrées including grains, vegetables, fruits, legumes, and rice. This section occupies the largest section of the triangle. It is the largest source of food in our world. Coincidently, it requires the least amount of energy for production.

The middle tier of the triangle contains members that eat from the bottom food tier – people, cows, goats, camels, giraffes and elephants. The top tier is the smallest. This tier eats from the middle tier. This tier includes predators such as hawks and cheetahs and lions. Humans that eat meat cross over into this tier.

Compare the abundance of energy required to produce a calf. Then consider the small amount of energy required to produce an equal amount of wheat. It requires much less energy, effort and time to produce a bundle of wheat than a calf equal in weight. The extra energy could have been used to create enough wheat to feed more people.

In theory, we could transfer all of the energy we devote to raising livestock to growing an increased amount of vegetation. We would ultimately have more food on Earth. The surplus of food could then be used to eliminate world hunger.

Giving up eating meat may not be desirable to you. But if you can, more power to you. Realistically, there are billions of people who enjoy a scrumptious meat dinner now and then. It would be easier for each of us to decrease the amount of meat we eat. Being a vegetarian just one day a week will ultimately make an impact on world hunger.

94.

THE "NO'S" OF NUTRITION

The two most common nutrition questions are "What is the worst thing I could eat?" and "What should I stay away from?" Here are the top three devastating nutritional health moves you can make.

1. Drinking more than two servings of a sugary beverage a day. This includes alcohol, soda, and punches.

Many do not realize the number of empty calories they put into their body each day. Some people have sugar-laden drinks by the hour. This is very unhealthy. Decreasing to one to two drinks per day will dramatically help you return to a desirable body weight. You could be short-changing yourself elsewhere in your diet if you haven't gained any weight from drinking these beverages. Do you wonder why you are tired all of the time? Perhaps you are anemic from lack of iron. Do you wonder why your back is hunched over at age thirty-six? You should have been consuming calcium rich beverages instead of soda pop.

2. Keeping snack and dessert food around the house

If it is not accessible or it's too hard make you will not be able to eat it for a snack. Make yourself work for favorite indulgences. Want a cookie? Make a batch and eat two. Give the rest to your neighbors. Need ice cream? Walk to the ice cream store. What if you *are* the neighbor receiving the batch of cookies? Wrap the cookies in foil, staple shut, stick in a plastic bag and freeze them.

3. Being out of energy balance buy either eating too much or not exercising enough or both.

Do you know if you are out of energy balance? It is likely you are out of energy balance when you are not at your ideal body weight range. Remember playing on the teeter-totters in elementary school? You were either weighting the totter down or you were high in the sky. Move yourself into balance by moderating your energy in with your energy out. The best way to check this is to compare your weight with your height. Insurance companies originally designed weight range charts after years of studies to determine the healthiest weight ranges. A person that is out of range can be more susceptible to disease. One out of every two Americans is out of their range.

If you are making all three mistakes, choose one at a time to concentrate on, change your life habits and then move on to the next. You will notice a change just from changing one of these.

95

THE SAGA CONTINUES

White-collar workers may have a degree or two to tout. However there is not much to brag about when it comes to how active they are. Most white-collar jobs are sedentary, with the exception of jobs requiring a lot of walking and traveling. We are more efficient. We are becoming fatter.

Weight maintenance is very simple. The amount of energy (calories in food) you consume must equal the amount of calories you expend. Compare it to a teeter-totter. Balancing the teeter-totter requires equal weight on both sides. The same goes for your body. Balancing your amount of activity with the amount of food you eat causes weight maintenance. Eating more energy than you are expending causes weight gain. Eating less energy (calories) than you expend causes weight loss.

Are you doing a weight-loss plan and not losing weight? You could be over estimating your activity level. Review your typical day. Is it spent sitting in front of a computer? Or is your workday filled with strenuous activities? Here are the different activity levels:

> **Very lightly active** – Seated or standing activities, artwork, driving, laboratory work, cooking, playing a musical instrument, computer/typing work, sewing, ironing, etc.

> **Lightly active** – Jobs requiring casual walking (3 mph), garage work, electrician jobs, carpentry, restaurant workers, housecleaning, teaching, golf, and sailing.

Moderately active – Gardening, cycling, skiing, dancing, tennis, walking while carrying a load.

Heavily active – Hiking, lumber-jacks, construction work, basketball, football and soccer.

Exceptional – Professional or Olympic athletes have exceptional activity levels.

What is your average activity level? You may need fewer calories than you think. Most Americans are lightly active.

96

RECIPE RECONSTRUCTION

Do you enjoy cooking? Maybe you are cooking less because of your hectic life. You should make an effort to cook once in a while. Eating out is a treat but dining in can be just as pleasurable. When the weekend comes take the opportunity to go to the grocery store, relax and cook a spectacular meal at home. You need to know the tricks to altering recipes to make them lower fat and lower calorie.

Accompany every meal with a tossed salad. You can skip adding the extras such as croutons, bacon bits, and cheese. Tossing salad greens, sliced tomato, and cucumber with a splash of vinegar and olive oil and pepper is the simplest way to go. Feeling adventurous? Try this easy vinaigrette made with a favorite flavoring, vanilla. Combine 1/4 c. olive oil, 1/3 c. vinegar, and 1 T. pure vanilla extract, 1/2 tsp. salt and 1/4 tsp. pepper. Whisk vigorously.

There are three different styles for cooking the main course:

Convenience - Many people are opting for the easiest cooking method. They open the package, place it in the microwave oven, and press the cook button! Choose frozen foods that have reduced fat or low fat.

Gourmet - Gourmet cooking can be time consuming. These entrees usually do not contain a plethora of added fat. Try doing this on weekends for a healthy change.

Family Style - Casseroles and one-dish meals occupy this category. They are often the choices you find at a church potluck or in the fundraiser cookbooks.

Family style cooking is delicious. However the recipes need to be "reconstructed" for better health. Don't trash the "Annual Fundraiser Cookbook". Practice these tips with a couple of the casseroles.

Most of these casseroles use a plethora of cheese. Cheese is a fine food to top casseroles with. However cheese adds a lot of saturated fat. There are some benefits though. Because of its calcium, it can help prevent osteoporosis. You can avert cardiovascular disease and osteoporosis simultaneously by using low fat cheese. Part-skim mozzarella is a fabulous low-fat cheese. Use this on your homemade pizzas and other Italian delights like manicotti and lasagna.

The next common ingredient found in casseroles adds the creamy texture to the dish. This could be another dairy product such as sour cream, a creamed soup, or mayonnaise. Opt for the low-fat or fat free version. Combined in a casserole the fat free flavor is undetectable. If you cannot stand the fat free after a couple tries, use low fat. People using low calorie or calorie-free counterparts are more likely to be within their appropriate weight range.

Does the casserole call for ground beef? Fool your family and substitute ground turkey. To truly receive the lowered fat content of poultry you must go with a product that reads "100% ground turkey meat". Anything else incorporates the poultry skin. If you go that route you might as well have had beef.

Sauces such as salsa, ketchup, enchilada sauce, mustard, steak sauce, and teriyaki sauce are fat free flavorings that do not need to be altered.

Sweets can range anywhere between muffins and coffeecakes to cookies. Can you have your cake and eat it too when it comes to reduced cooking? Yes you can. Try not to eat more than one serving. Some people have a lack of control when faced with reduced versions. These people would have been better off having one serving of the regular version rather than ten of the low-fat food! Here are some other substitutes:

Food	Substitute
Oil	Applesauce
Butter	Yogurt
Whole Milk	Skim Milk
Eggs	Egg Substitute or Egg Whites
White Flour	Whole Wheat Flour

You will not believe how many calories you can save by reconstructing recipes. Engage in taste tests with your family. Test two types of cornbread. Make the first with whole eggs, whole milk and white flour. On the revamped version substitute egg whites, skim milk, and whole-wheat flour. Reducing the fat will allow the other flavors to be enhanced. You might find that the majority of your family will prefer the healthier version.

97.

BODY MOBILES

You must take care of your car whether you have a Porsche or an old Buick. Your car lasts longer the better you maintain it. Do you take your car to the hand car wash weekly? Do you make sure it gets it an oil change every 3000 miles? What is the point of all of the attention your car receives? Maybe it enhances the pride you hold for your prized possession. It could be that you want to retain good value. Or you may just want to attract a member of the opposite sex. Be what it may, your car is an important aspect of your life. It gets you around! However, your car will never by as important as your own body! Your body will carry you places even when a car fails you. You should give your body the same respect you have for your other prized possessions.

Are you convinced? You run on food, your car runs on fuel. You can't "go" without putting the necessary ingredients in either one. You must use quality fuel however! You'd never fill your car tank with diesel fuel. Your car would not go too far. Then why do you fill your body with ingredients that cause you to break down -   cardiovascular disease, Type 2 Diabetes, stroke or diverticulitis? You would fill your car with premium gasoline if you were smart. You would also eat a well-balanced diet.

Some busy folk argue that they don't have time to eat healthy. They grab fast food for dinner to save time. These people will later spend all of the saved time at the hospital. Some people are too busy to fill their tanks with gas. They run on empty, and on occasion, they run out of gas. No time was saved. In either case these people are being careless in order to save time. Eating healthy takes only a couple extra minutes a day.

"Service maintenance... Service maintenance..." your light on your car blinks. It is time to get an oil change. Better take it in for its regular tune up. While you're at it, make an appointment for a health check-up with your doctor. Get your blood taken to access your cholesterol, triglycerides and HDL's. Your doctor will test your blood sugar, checking for Type 2 Diabetes and other diseases evident by a blood sample. It is important to check-up your body's health regularly. You can prevent a problem before it becomes out of control. Similarly a mechanic might recommend replacing your brakes for fear they might give out soon. It is just as vital to catch your high blood pressure before the mortal stroke paralyzes you for half a year.

Have you ever had an automobile battery go dead? You turn the key and nothing happens. Frustrating isn't it? Especially if a mechanic told you it was time to replace it. Then why do you insist on plopping down on the couch every night in front of the television when you know you should be exercising? Move, will you? At least exercise in *front* of the television. You can exercise in front of the TV by doing yoga poses, sit-ups, push-ups and healthy stretches. Make it a priority every day to achieve some movement in your life. Garden, walk to the grocery store, play with your kids, dance, basketball, *whatever*... just move!

Some people insist, "I don't have time for exercise!" You will face hassle by neglecting to exercise. And believe me; your stay at the hospital due to your heart attack is going to take much more time, scrutiny, effort and money than replacing a dead car battery. When you exercise you are adding time to your life.

Treat your body as you would your most prized possession. Your body *is* your most prized possession. If you take the same care of your body as you do with your car, you will live a long and mobile life.

98.

AMERICA UNDER ATTACK

September 11, 2001 was the most horrific day of our lives. The amount of pain and suffering that occurred as a result of that tragedy spread rapidly in the hearts of people across the United States. Our moral minds cannot fathom that many people dying consecutively. There is always good in every occurrence and I am determined to find good in this one. Our value of life has changed.

Because we value life more we should not ignore one "attacker" we are more vulnerable to than terrorists. Compare the number of people who died on 9-11 to the number who die from another attack. It is called heart attack. Let's use Orange County, California for example. Orange County is a place where people are health-conscious and active. The number of deaths in Orange County alone due to heart attack in 1997 was 5152 people.

People die everyday from heart attacks. We have become desensitized. It is a part of our American culture. We eat extra large sized meals at fast food joints with no activity for days, even weeks. This is the planning process of the attack.

After some time passes, a health professional warns you of a possible attack in your future. The clues are there, you are over weight and your results from your blood show high levels of low density lipoproteins (the bad fats). You ignore the signs of the attack all the while thinking, "It will not happen to me." You go on with your life continuing to eat the same while postponing your exercising once again. Then it happens, one dreaded day in your life, the attack! It is a devastating day for you. The rest of America continues living, bringing *themselves* closer to their attack.

It is a sickening reality but it is true. This form of attack kills more than any terrorist has ever planned. In America, every thirty-three seconds, someone experiences a heart attack. Do the math. That is 2618 attacks per day and a grand 955,563 per year.

You need to have the same spirit for your body's health as you had for your country during the week of September 11, 2001. Lace up some tennis shoes and become active. This is your first step toward a healthy heart. The American Heart Association has identified risks you take to make yourself vulnerable to heart disease. Being inactive is one of them. Smoking is another major risk factor for heart disease. Fresh produce, seafood and whole grains are all foods that are fantastic deterrents of heart disease. Eating these foods is like putting a "health army" in your body. These foods are proven to fight the building blocks of heart attack. If you are eating healthy and exercising, chances are you are within your proper weight range. Maintaining a healthy weight saves your heart a significant amount of stress.

This is a serious health epidemic that you need to take control of. There is no better way to begin then with your self today. Eat in moderation, exercise, quit smoking and de-stress yourself. Eliminate the number one killer of America!

99.

I FEEL HUNGRY, THEREFORE I EAT

The new trend in dieting is intuitive eating. Intuitive eating does not involve planned menus or fat gram and calorie counting. It isn't weekly weight checks and hundreds of dollars either. Intuitive eating is as simple as eating when you are hungry. This is a concept that is foreign to many of us avid dieters. We are more familiar with depriving ourselves when we are famished and eating when we are not hungry. Though to most of us dieting seems to be the answer to weight loss, it obviously is not effective enough. Ninety percent of dieters regain lost weight within only five years. With that in mind, health professionals and dietitians are turning to a new answer, intuitive eating.

Remember when you were a child? After eating breakfast, you could not wait to go outside and play. Food was a distant thought in your mind, not an obsession like it is now for some of us. While you played you were focused completely on what you were playing. What time was lunch? That just depended on when you became hungry. Sometimes you were hungry at around eleven in the morning, other days you were not hungry until 1 – 1:30 p.m. What did you choose to eat? Some days you were slightly hungry so a peanut butter and jelly sandwich was enough. But those days when you were starving, you accompanied that sandwich with a glass of grape juice and a handful of potato chips. As a child you were a great example of intuitive eating. Where did that healthy mindset go? It was lost years ago when dieting, weight and food became an obsession. It is never too late to bring this eating pattern back into your lifestyle.

Begin by trashing all diet books, except this one! There are no rigid rules to intuitive eating so those books will be of no use to you.

Accept the fact that some days you will not have the perfect diet. In the long run your nutrient intake will balance out.

Be in tune with your body before, during and after you eat. Ask yourself, "Am I really physically hungry?" Rate you hunger on a scale of one to ten: one being extremely hungry, ten being uncomfortably full. Aim to keep yourself around ratings three to seven. This way you will refrain from uncontrollable eating. If you are trying to lose weight, keep yourself around ratings two to six. If you want to gain weight, shoot for four to eight.

Eliminate your stereotypes of food. There is no "good" or "bad" food when you eat intuitively. All foods are allowed within moderation. For example: eating cheesecake everyday is not moderation.

With intuitive eating there is one rule and one rule only. Eat when you are hungry. It's that simple.

100.

TWO RULES TO LIVE BY

The amount of information about nutrition and health is overwhelming. It is difficult to know what is valid and what is not. There are two basic rules for healthy eating. Validate all information you absorb with these two rules. (Exception: if you are a person with an existing medical problem these rules may not apply to you).

Rule #1 – All foods are good in moderation! Not one single food is "bad" for you. A diet is legit if and only if it allows for you to eat all foods in moderation. Even cheesecake is allowed in a healthy moderate diet. It may not be a piece of cheesecake everyday or a large piece like you wish. Once a week, a very small piece after a Sunday night dinner is a good example of moderation. Eliminating carbohydrates from your diet is not eating in moderation.

Rule #2 – Eat to live instead of living to eat! Why do we eat? Eating is essential to live. Think of eating as a way to fuel and nourish the body. Want to know if you are eating to live? It can best be determined by examining the reason you are eating. Is it hunger, boredom, stress or maybe pleasure? Hunger should be the answer ninety percent of the time. The other ten percent should be light eating in social situations. Let's say it is your birthday. Someone at the office baked you a cake. It is polite to eat one piece. But if you have a second and you are not hungry, then you are breaking the rule.

Follow these two rules for the rest of your life. There is no list of foods you need to remember to avoid. There is no combination of foods that are good or bad to eat. There is not one food that is a miracle worker. Just remember that all foods fit into a healthy diet and only eat when you are hungry. Simple as that!

DEEP THOUGHTS FROM THE NUTRITION EXPERTS

A dietitian is your best source for nutritional advice. I've collaborated with some of my colleagues to provide you with thoughts we would like you to use in your life:

> Do not get too hungry. People who get too hungry want carrot cake, not carrots; apple pie, not apples.
>
> **Nancy Clark, M.S., R.D.**

. . . .

> To save tons of calories at a Mexican restaurant, bring your own baked tortilla chips, ask for an empty basket, load up on the salsa, and nibble away guiltlessly!
>
> **Merrin Folender, R.D.**

. . . .

> Choose whole foods. Select foods with the least amount of processing such as fresh fruits and vegetables, small amounts of lean meats, fish or chicken and whole grain products.
>
> **Johanna Donnenfield, M.S., R.D.**

Most people want to lose *body fat* weight, which means including daily physical activity and eating anything you *really enjoy* less often.

Name withheld

. . . .

Being a vegan, vegetarian myself, I would suggest a more vegetarian cuisine; a cornucopia of fresh produce, a variety of different beans, omega 3 fatty acids, fish, nuts, seeds, soy milk, fruit and variety of herbs, spices and flavors. Include different tastes: sweet, bitter, pungent, sour and astringent. Decrease salt and fried fatty foods. Our bodies and minds are influenced by our choices. Make eating a spiritual experience and prepare food with love. Discover the deeper mystery of foods and those that create harmony in your body. Remember that *food* is your energy supply.

Barbara Beznos, R.D., L.D.

. . . .

Our metabolism works most efficiently when we eat small, frequent meals throughout they day. Wait no longer than three to four hours between each meal and include a serving of carbohydrates, fat and protein.

Theresa DeLorenzo, R.D.

Most Americans are afraid of food, fear of fat, fear of carbohydrates, should I eat more protein or less? Americans have been following weight loss and fad diets for over forty years and without much success. It's time to return to eating *real* foods, those foods that are as close to the way they are grown. The healthy eating message has not changed at all, five to nine servings of vegetables and fruits, low saturated fat protein and vegetable protein, and whole grains, breads and cereals. Along with healthy eating should be a healthy dose of movement, dare we say exercise, each day. Include fruits and vegetables with each meal, start with fruit, it's easy to carry and enjoyed by all.

Don Mankie, R.D.

. . . .

Managing one's weight is not done with dieting, but it begins from the inside. Getting in touch with your levels of hunger and fullness will conquer weight. Dieting involves tuning out the very thing we need to listen to: our appetite.

Cindy Sims, R.D.

Eat it all if it is small! Be happy with less! Buy single servings of food! 1 scoop of ice cream. 1 donut! I tell my clients about my visiting relatives from Italy. They found the portions so big they split their meals when we ate out. When you dine out cut your portions in half!

Name Withheld

. . . .

By removing *just* a spoonful of *every* food item on your plate, *every* time you eat, you can lose up to four pounds per week.

Dr. Susan Shapiro, R.D.

. . . .

For the compulsive overeater:

1. Stop
2. Think
3. React

Stop and rate your hunger level. One through ten. One starving, five contentment, and ten stuffed.

Think about what you are really feeling in terms of emotions. i.e. sad, lonely, angry, tired

Reach appropriately. Follow through with the planned escape food item, call a support person up, or write about those emotions

Name Withheld

. . . .

Health equals balance: take time to nourish your body with five fruits and vegetables, exercise moderately for you body and mind, and take time to relax and reflect everyday.

Amber Pawlowski, R.D.

LEGAL NOTICE

Atkins Diet is a registered trademark of Atkins Nutritions, Inc. Deal-A-Meal is a registered trademark of Richard Simmons, Inc. Weight Watchers is a registered trademark of Weight Watchers International, Inc. Slim Fast is a registered trademark of Slim Fast Foods Corporation.

Other brand, product and company names are trademarks of their respective owners. The materials contained herein are summary in nature, subject to change, and intended for general information only.

SUGGESTED READING

MacIntyre J. Facts Of Life. Spirit, 9:10, 2000.
Susan L. Burke, MS, RD, CDE
Manager of Nutrition Support
Burke, Susan L. ediets.com

Gershoff, Stanley. Did you know...
Tufts University Health & Nutrition Letter, 16:2, 1998.

Gershoff, Stanley. Is Organic More Nutritious?
Tuft University Health & Nutrition Letter, 15:7, 1997.

Mendelsohn, Susan Joy. Psy.D.,
Dr. Ediets.com, Jan. 4, 2001.

SR Rolfes and EN Whitney. Planning A Healthy Diet..
Understanding Nutrition. 7th ed., eds.
P Lewis.(Los Angeles: West Publishing Company, 1996), p46.

LK Mahan & S Escott-Stump. Nutritional Care in Intestinal Disease.
Krause's Food, Nutrition, & Diet Therapy 9th ed, eds D Ruth, BN Cullen
and M Connor. (Philadelphia: W.B. Saunders Company) 615-6.

Rosenberg, I. More People Lifting Weights – and Getting Injured.
Tuft University Health & Nutrition Letter, 18:9; 2000.

H McCord & G McVeigh. Drinker's Formula Could Save Your Life.
Prevention, Vol. 53: No. 1, 2001.

Gershoff, S. Alcohol's Role in Breast Cancer Quantified.
Tufts University Health & Nutrition Letter, 16:2, 1998.

Gershoff, S. Reducing Breast Cancer Risk.
Tufts University Healthy & Nutrition Letter, 15:11, 1998.

Landry G. Fitness Guru's 24 Great Reasons To Exercise.
Ediets.com, Jan. 16, 2001.

Giddens J, Krug SK, Tsang R, Guo S, Miodovnik M, Prada J. Pregnant
adolescent and adult women have similarly low intakes of selected nutrients.
J Am Diet Assoc, 100:11, 2000.

SR Rolfes and EN Whitney. Life Cycle Nutrition: Pregnancy and Lactation.
Understanding Nutrition 7th ed, eds P Lewis (Los Angeles: West Publishing
Company, 1996). P554-558.

Waterhouse D. Like Mother, Like Daughter.
Waterhouse Publishing

Gershoff, S. Outpacing Middle-Age Spread.
Tuft University Health & Nutrition Letter, 16:9, 1998.

Exercise Assesment.
NutriWay Cholesterol and Weight Control Program. 1998.

SR Rolfes and EN Whitney. Life Cycle Nutrition: Adulthood and the Later
Years. Understanding Nutrition 7th ed.eds P Lewis (Los Angeles: West
Publishing Company, 1996). P621.

Bidlack W. Functional Foods to Enhance Health.
Foods for the Future Conference.
The California Dietetic Association, Orange District, Jan. 20, 2001.

Picking Organic. Albertsons Food & Drug. Albertson's

http://www.akbar.com/Bookont3.htm. Project on Black Teas and It's
Health Benefits.
Tea Exporters Directory 1996 August 13, 2001.

http://www.usaweekend.com/01_issues/010204/010204eatsmart.html.
"Chocolate Lovers, Take Heart"
USAWeekend.com February 4, 2001.

Hudepohl, D. 26 Live-Healthy Lessons From Around the World.
Self, August 2001.

Thayer, S. "Monitoring Chronic Diseases in Orange County.
A Report Based on Chronic Disease and Hospitalizations in 1997."
June 2000.

Post, Elizabeth L. Emily Post's Etiquette 15th ed.
HarperCollins Publishers United States of America 1992.

OCDA month meeting,
January 2001.

http://www.usaweekend.com/health/carper_archive/950813eat_smart_to
matoes.html. "Tomatoes Secret Strenght".
USA Weekend.com August 11-13, 1995.

Rich, T. http://www.jewfaq.org/food.htm.
"Jewish Cooking".

Stern, MP, K Williams and SM Haffner.
http://www.annals.org/issues/v136n8/fpdf/200204160-00002.pdf.
"Identification of Persons at High-Risk for Type 2 Diabetes Mellitus:
Do we Need the Oral Glucose Tolerance Test?"
Annals of Internal Medicine. Vol 136. April 16, 2002.. PP 575-581.

Diabetes Disparities Among Racial and Ethnic Minorities. November 2001.
AHRQ Publication No. 02-P007.
Agency for Healthcare Research and Quality, Rockville, MD.
http://www.ahrq.gov/research/diabdisp.htm

American Heart Association, 2002 Heart and Stroke Statistical Update.
Dallas, Texas: American Heart Assocation, 2001.

National Cancer Institute. Cancer Health Disparities.Bethesda,
Maryland. April 21, 2002.
http://newscenter.cancer.gov/pressreleases/healthdisparities.html.

Reuters Health. Gene Variations Linked To Lung Cancer Risk.
New York. May 1, 2002.
http://www.nlm.nih.gov/medlineplus/news/fullstory_7393.html

Osteoporosis. May 15, 2002.
http://www.nlm.nih.gov/medlineplus/ency/article/000360.htm#causesAn
dRisk

Testicular Cancer.January 26, 2001.
http://www.nlm.nih.gov/medlineplus/ency/article/001288.htm#causesAndRisk

Sandrick, K. Zoo Nutrition: A Walk on the Wild Side.
J Am Diet Assoc, Vol. 101:8, 2001.

Pearlstinc, N. Loss Leaders. In Style, Spring 2002.
Fitness, March 2002.

Johnson DB, D Eaton, P Wahl, C Gleason.
Public Health Nutrition Practice in the United States.
J Am Diet Assoc.2001;101: 529-534.

Osteoporosis Online. September 13, 2002
http://www.osteoporosis.ca/OSTEO/D02-01c.html#maximize

Caffeine and Bone Density and Older Women, September 13, 2002
http://www.eatright.com/erm/erm010802.html

Caffeine and Migraines. October 27, 2002
http://www.batnet.com/spencer/faq1.html#19

Veena and Neena – Indian Dances. November 17, 2002.
http://bellytwins.com/default2.htm.

Lawhon C, E Terry. Twisted Sisters. In Style, November 2002.

ISBN 155395560-9